Advance Praise for *Overdiagnosis in Psychiatry*

"Dr. Paris is a psychiatrist who knows his onions and so can make you weep. He weeps at the failure to recognize strengths in people rather than weaknesses, and after reading his book we should all gain from one of its key sentences 'it would probably be better to define mental health, not as happiness, but as resilience in the face of adversity.'"

—**Peter Tyrer, Professor of Community Psychiatry, Centre for Mental Health, Imperial College, London**

"Most discussions of diagnosis focus on problems with missed diagnoses or misdiagnosis. Dr. Paris does the field a great favor by focusing on the problem of overdiagnosis, and showing how it is as great a problem as underdiagnosis."

—**Mark Zimmerman, Professor of Psychiatry and Human Behavior, Brown Medical School, Providence, RI**

"Too much medicine can be bad for your health—overdiagnosis and over-treatment are now serious public health problems. Dr Paris has provided an important pebble in the David vs Goliath battle to contain the medical-industrial complex."

—**Allen Frances, Professor Emeritus and former Chair, Duke University and author of *Saving Normal*, Coronado, CA**

"Dr. Joel Paris has written a wonderfully provocative book that will irritate some readers and delight others. With opinions based on his many years working in the trenches, Dr. Paris points out the problems of overdiagnosis, misdiagnose, and diagnostic epidemics that have been fueled in part by overenthusiasm for the DSM. Written in an accessible style, this book is bound to become a classic in the field."

—**Donald W. Black, MD, Professor, Department of Psychiatry, University of Iowa Roy J. and Lucille A. Carver College of Medicine, Iowa City, IA**

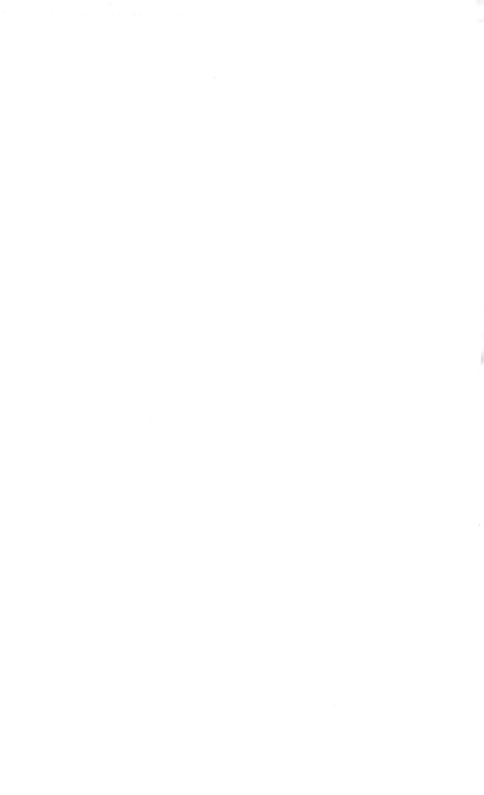

OVERDIAGNOSIS IN PSYCHIATRY

How Modern Psychiatry Lost Its Way While Creating a Diagnosis for Almost All of Life's Misfortunes

JOEL PARIS, MD

Professor of Psychiatry, McGill University

OXFORD
UNIVERSITY PRESS

Oxford University Press is a department of the University of
Oxford. It furthers the University's objective of excellence in research,
scholarship, and education by publishing worldwide.

Oxford   New York
Auckland   Cape Town   Dar es Salaam   Hong Kong   Karachi
Kuala Lumpur   Madrid   Melbourne   Mexico City   Nairobi
New Delhi   Shanghai   Taipei   Toronto

With offices in
Argentina   Austria   Brazil   Chile   Czech Republic   France   Greece
Guatemala   Hungary   Italy   Japan   Poland   Portugal   Singapore
South Korea   Switzerland   Thailand   Turkey   Ukraine   Vietnam

Oxford is a registered trademark of Oxford University Press
in the UK and certain other countries.

Published in the United States of America by
Oxford University Press
198 Madison Avenue, New York, NY 10016

Library of Congress Cataloging-in-Publication Data
Paris, Joel, 1940–, author.
Overdiagnosis in psychiatry: how modern psychiatry lost its way while
creating a diagnosis for almost all of life's misfortunes/Joel Paris.
    p. ; cm.
ISBN 978-0-19-935064-3 (alk. paper)
I. Title.
[DNLM: 1. Mental Disorders—diagnosis.   2. Diagnostic Errors.
3. Diagnostic Techniques and Procedures—utilization. WM 141]
RC473.D54
616.89′075—dc23
2014039665

9 8 7 6 5 4 3 2 1
Printed in the United States of America
on acid-free paper

This book is dedicated to my fellow researchers in psychiatry, who have taught me the importance of caution in clinical practice.

CONTENTS

PART III. DIAGNOSIS AND NORMALITY

ACKNOWLEDGMENTS

Don Black and Mark Zimmerman read earlier versions of this book and made many helpful suggestions for its improvement.

INTRODUCTION

WHAT HAPPENED TO PSYCHIATRY?

Psychiatry has lost its soul. I am heartsick at what has happened to the profession I love. Overdiagnosis moves lock-step with over-treatment with drugs, ignoring the life circumstances of the patients we treat. Psychiatrists have forgotten the listening skills and careful attention to clinical phenomena that once made their specialty unique. I have written this book for mental health practitioners, for patients, and for the many members of the public who are interested in the fate of psychiatry. They will want to know how and why we got into this kind of trouble.

I always used to say I loved psychiatry because it was about life. I now realize this is not true. Psychopathology does not define the human condition. I worry about the dangers of confusing unhappiness with mental illness. That was the error made by a previous generation of psychodynamic psychiatrists whose theories claimed to account not only for symptoms, but for all of normal psychology. Now the same mistake is being made again, this time by biological psychiatrists who promote an expansion of the boundaries of diagnosis.

Modern psychiatry has rejected its long-standing psychosocial perspective, and has adopted a narrow version of the medical model. From the National Institute of Mental Health (NIMH) to the National Association for the Mentally Ill (NAMI), the motto has been adopted that mental disorders are brain diseases. This dogma is half-true and half-untrue. Yes, everything we observe clinically also happens in the brain. But you cannot understand the mind on that basis alone.

A landmark event occurred in 1980, when the American Psychiatric Association adopted the third edition of the *Diagnostic and Statistical Manual of Mental Disorders* (*DSM-III*), a system that became standard all over the world. Over the next several decades, the *DSM*, including its 1994 revision as *DSM-IV*, was the primary tool used by psychiatrists to classify mental illness, both in the United States and around the world. The *DSM* system is now in its fifth edition (*DSM-5*), and while there have been a few changes, it remains essentially the same. It describes almost any type of psychological symptom using hundreds of categories that include everything from distress and disappointment to disabling illness. The *DSM* makes many of life's misfortunes diagnosable, and implicitly offers psychiatry as a cure for unhappiness.

Paradoxically, one would have thought that psychiatry's move back into the medical mainstream would have encouraged it to focus on severe mental illnesses. That would have been logical, given the many patients who absolutely need specialist care. But psychiatrists working in outpatient settings, community clinics, or private offices see patients who are much less ill. They want their work to be validated (and made insurable) by the diagnostic system. This is why *DSM-5* encourages clinicians to give every patient a psychiatric diagnosis (for which they can be reimbursed). In this way, economic factors have made the temptation to medicalize the human condition almost irresistible.

The most distressing change in psychiatry is the way it is now being practiced. Patients are often seen for 10–15 minutes, and are given little time to talk about what is happening in their lives. Diagnoses are made rapidly—and often inaccurately. Instead of listening, and asking about current circumstances, psychiatrists focus on a checklist of symptoms, a kind of parody of the criteria listed in the *DSM* manual. Based on the answers to these questions, prescriptions will be written for almost every problem—and "adjusted" every time a patient comes in feeling distressed. It is also worth noting that the practice of psychiatry becomes more lucrative when more patients are seen briefly (and sent off with prescriptions). This way of working meets with approval from psychiatrists and other professionals who believe that mental illness is entirely due to molecules that have gone awry. It is also good news for pharmaceutical companies, whose profits depend on the high volume of drugs prescribed for the most common mental disorders.

For all these reasons, I have become critical of the way many of my colleagues practice psychiatry. But these errors are not based on malignant intent. My colleagues believe they are doing the best for patients, and that talking and listening are old-fashioned practices that belong to an unenlightened past. They want to do *something* for every patient, even when there is no scientific basis for doing so. They also live in a social environment that strongly reinforces these practices.

The result is a serious overdiagnosis of mental disorders, leading to a serious over-treatment of patients. I have written this book to counter that trend. I want to send out a message that psychiatry is over-stretched. Instead of prescribing treatment for what Freud once called "normal human unhappiness," we need to focus our efforts on patients who are seriously ill, and who need us the most. We do not need to diagnose the human condition.

OVERDIAGNOSIS IN MEDICINE

Psychiatry is not the only field of medicine suffering from a tendency to medicalize life's viccissitudes. One strand is what Moynihan et al. (2002) called "disease mongering," that is, considering normal variations to be pathological and treating them as illnesses. This radical expansion of medicine and the resulting overdiagnosis reflect a number of factors, including the wish of physicians to expand their domain, the wish of patients to find help for suffering, and massive propaganda from the pharmaceutical industry. The danger is that over-zealous diagnosis fails to help the sick while harming the healthy.

Another reason for overdiagnosis is the wish to identify and treat illness in its early stages. This has long been a goal of specialists in cancer, who have supported large public programs to encourage people to be screened, using procedures such as mammography or the measurement of prostate-specific antigen (PSA). Even though these procedures have had at best mixed results, most physicians think it is better to screen than not to screen. The same idea is held by most patients.

In psychiatry, similar ideas have gained a good deal of traction. The principle has been applied to depression, for which mass screening tests have sometimes been carried out. Unfortunately, such measures pick up distress, not treatable disease, and do not assess severity. By pathologizing episodes that would resolve on their own, screening can do more harm than good (Thombs et al., 2008). Similarly, the movement for the recognition of early psychosis (McGorry et al., 2010) runs against a similar problem: people with subclinical symptoms do not necessarily go on to develop full disorders.

Overdiagnosis in medicine unnecessarily worries people, and often leads to futile and ineffective treatment. Perhaps its greatest problem is that it diverts resources away from the seriously ill, who need our care the most, and directs them to people who are either not ill or who can be expected to recover from their symptoms without treatment. Psychiatrists have enough work to do without expanding the boundaries of the disorders into the world of the "worried well" or of people going through a "bad patch."

Life would be simpler if we could establish a clear definition of mental disorder, and separate it from normal unhappiness. But as Allen Frances (2013) has observed, doing so has proven almost impossible. Each edition of the DSM has attempted to provide such a definition, but each definition requires a subjective judgment as to what is illness and what are the vicissitudes of the human condition. This has made it easier to medicalize problems of living.

DON'T BLAME THE *DSM-5*!

To what extent is the *DSM* system responsible for the current plight of psychiatry and the overdiagnosis of mental disorders? With the publication of *DSM-5*, critics of psychiatry had a field day criticizing its diagnostic system. Insiders, such as Allen Frances (2013), focused on retaining the concept of normality, and not expanding psychiatric diagnosis to people who are, like the rest of us, struggling with their lives. Outsiders, such as the psychotherapist Gary Greenberg (2013), have used problems with *DSM-5* as a platform to attack the credibility of psychiatry as a discipline.

My own view, developed in a previous book (Paris, 2013), is that we need to view *DSM-5* in a broader context. It is not fair to hold the latest edition to account for trends that have changed, and continue to change, the very nature of psychiatry. A diagnostic manual is a tool that can be applied in different ways. Used cautiously, it need not lead to overdiagnosis or over-treatment. Nor does the *DSM* force us to focus on symptoms to the exclusion of understanding our patients and their life histories.

Psychiatrists in practice, anxious to be "real doctors," have adopted an ideology based on neuroscience (Paris, 2008a). The belief that mental disorders are "nothing but" brain diseases, strongly influenced by the pharmaceutical industry, is the source of the problem. Psychiatrists do not write most of the prescriptions that patients receive—family doctors and internists do. But as specialists, psychiatrists have great influence on primary care. Family doctors who consult with us are very likely to be told to prescribe more drugs, not less. I sometimes think I am the only one writing consultations suggesting that patients are being over-medicated and that psychotherapy has not been seriously considered.

When *DSM-III* was introduced in 1980, I was a strong supporter of the new system. I had learned *DSM-I* in medical school and *DSM-II* in residency. Like most psychiatrists, I was unimpressed with the theoretical validity and the sloppy definitions in these early editions. Moreover, psychiatrists couldn't even agree about the most basic diagnoses. With no gold standard, patients might see three psychiatrists and receive three different opinions. To attain scientific credibility, the classification system needed to become more reliable. While disagreements still occur, the reason does not lie with the way the *DSM* editions have been written. Practitioners make diagnoses intuitively, and rarely follow the guidelines in the *DSM* very closely (Zimmerman and Galione, 2010).

Even in *DSM-5*, the reliability of diagnosis remains problematic, as shown by the disappointing results of recent field trials (Regier et al., 2013). Moreover, the categories listed in the manual have uncertain validity, in that all diagnoses are entirely based on signs and symptoms, without confirmation from biomarkers. In that respect, *DSM-5* is no different from its predecessors. This was not a choice, but a necessity. Unlike the rest of medicine, psychiatry has no biological markers to validate *any* of its diagnostic categories.

It is possible to practice effective medicine without biomarkers, particularly in syndromes (such as migraine) that are not well understood. Moreover, psychiatry does as well as most medical specialties in getting its patients better (Leucht et al., 2012). But it is not yet able to ground clinical observations in objectively measured data. Biomarkers could, with time, guide physicians to the mechanisms behind illness. They would not answer all our questions, but if we had them, overdiagnosis would be a little less likely. Also, at this point, the causes of mental disorder remain largely unknown. That is why clinical diagnosis remains imprecise and uncertain. We cannot blame *DSM-5* for that problem. The manual simply reflects the imperfect state of our knowledge.

DIAGNOSTIC EPIDEMICS

A lack of knowledge should make psychiatrists cautious about their threshold for identifying mental disorders. Yet over recent decades, our field has developed an enthusiasm for making even *more* diagnoses, with an inflated prevalence that leads to *diagnostic epidemics.* Using current definitions (or expanded versions of existing categories), common mental disorders have become ubiquitous.

Frances (2013) has usefully documented how some diagnoses in psychiatry have doubled, tripled, or quadrupled in prevalence over recent years. For example, at least half the population can expect to suffer sometime in their life from what the *DSM* defines as "major depression" (Moffit et al., 2009). But these high numbers may only be an artifact of the way we make this diagnosis. The problem goes back decades, as psychiatry has adopted an overly inclusive definition of depression. It is difficult to say what the real prevalence of depression is when the concept of mood disorder is conflated with unhappiness.

Recently, three disorders traditionally considered to occur rather infrequently (bipolar disorder, attention deficit hyperactivity disorder [ADHD], and post-traumatic stress disorder [PTSD]) are being much more frequently diagnosed. Even disorders once considered quite rare (such as autism) are now being identified in large numbers of patients.

These changes in diagnostic practice tell us more about diagnostic fashion than about scientific progress. Diagnostic fads simply relabel patients that psychiatrists have always seen. The new categories are designed to either suggest a treatment option (as in bipolarity and ADHD), and/or to classify symptoms in the framework of disorders that are either a subject of clinical interest (as in PTSD) or that become eligible to more extensive treatment when identified (as in autism).

There are real dangers to diagnostic epidemics. All too often, they lead to incorrect and unnecessary treatment. Moreover, expansion of diagnosis to subclinical and non-clinical phenomena compromises the validity of the classification system. Finally, enthusiasm for making diagnoses prevents psychiatrists from separating psychopathology from normality. Major depression is the best example: 11% of the general population is currently taking antidepressants (Pratt et al., 2011)—a rate that is much higher than the prevalence of the disorders for which these drugs are usually prescribed. It has also been shown that prescriptions of these agents are often given for "off-label" indications (Mojtabai and Olfson, 2011).

There is no shortcut around these problems. Without a gold standard, screening instruments and scales can only have provisional validity. Psychiatric diagnosis is at best a common language, and current categories should not be treated as "real." This book will underline the difficulties in reaching accurate diagnoses, the dangers of overdiagnosing disorders, and the over-treatment of patients that follows from overdiagnosis, as well as the problems in recognizing what is normal.

PART I

BACKGROUND

DIAGNOSIS IN PSYCHIATRY

WHAT DIAGNOSIS IS—AND WHAT IT ISN'T

Medicine is an applied science that requires a classification of the phenomena it studies and treats. The features of illness also need to be described in a logical and scientific way. But the classification of disease does not have the same level of precision as six quarks or 92 natural chemical elements. We can more usefully compare illnesses to species in biology, which tend to be fuzzy at the edges and overlap with each other.

Diagnoses should ideally be based on specific pathological processes related to specific etiological pathways. The term *endophenotype* refers to the mechanisms that underlie disease—as opposed to *phenotypes*, clinical features that can be directly observed. Only some diseases in medicine have identifiable endophenotypes. Even so, diagnoses serve several functions. They guide medical research, allowing for the study of causes, prevalence, outcome, and methods of treatment. They serve as shorthand communication between professionals. Finally, they help patients, by providing an explanation for how and why they are ill.

Symptoms, when they cluster together, form syndromes. But without a specific etiology, syndromes are not diseases.

Since most mental illnesses remain syndromes, psychiatry describes its categories as "disorders." In other words, they do not qualify as diseases in the same way that most medical conditions do. We sometimes forget that mental disorders are convenient labels that lack any ultimate degree of reality.

Moreover, diagnosis in medicine should not be used to describe single symptoms, which can have many different causes. A good example of this mistake was a proposal (not, in the end, adopted) to create a separate category for suicidality in the fifth edition of the *Diagnostic and Statistical Manual of Mental Disorders (DSM-5)*. Any symptom can be described using standard scales, but unless symptoms reflect common mechanisms, they don't belong in a diagnostic manual. Finally, diagnosis should not be a political or a social statement. We should not diagnose post-traumatic stress disorder (PTSD) just because we sympathize with suffering in patients.

Overdiagnosis is usually the result of enthusiasm or zealotry, for either a theoretical concept or a treatment method. But expanding illness categories undermines the very purpose of classifying psychopathology. If diagnoses are blended into a spectrum, the differences between them are obscured, and research into their causes will be hobbled. The *DSM-5* system tried to define fewer diagnoses than *DSM-IV*, but still has too many. At this point we know too little to reduce this number by defining meaningful disease "spectra."

THE CURRENT STATE OF PSYCHIATRIC DIAGNOSIS

Medicine works best when accurate diagnosis leads to effective treatment. In contrast, overdiagnosis derives from inaccuracies that lead to ineffective or harmful treatment. Mistaken therapy is inevitable when we treat people with one problem as if they have another, and when people who are normal or have mild symptoms receive interventions that have been tested on severely ill patients.

In spite of its lack of knowledge of mechanisms, psychiatry has quite a few effective treatments. The effect sizes for our pharmacological interventions compare well to the rest of medicine (Leucht et al., 2012), and clinical trials demonstrate that many forms of psychotherapy are effective (Lambert, 2013). In general, the sickest patients almost always need pharmacotherapy, while mild to moderately ill patients often do as well or better with well-structured forms of psychotherapy. Yet all too often, we treat patients *only* with drugs, even when they don't respond to them and don't need them. This trend, which now dominates clinical practice (Mojtabai and Olfson, 2008), is based on the old saw that when you have a hammer, everything looks like a nail. Ideally, diagnosis should help us to distinguish patients who need pharmacotherapy from those in which its use is either doubtful or optional. But that is not what is happening. Instead, drug treatment for every patient is rationalized by the overuse of existing diagnostic categories.

Ultimately, diagnosis in psychiatry must be based on a better understanding of why people fall ill. We are just not there yet. In the past, psychiatry subscribed to a biopsychosocial model (Engel, 1980), in which multiple factors (biological, psychological, and social) were taken into account, both in etiology and in treatment. This model has been replaced by a reductionistic approach in which mental disorders are "nothing but" brain disorders. Leaders in psychiatric research want to redefine the specialty as a branch of neurology whose practice consists of "applied neuroscience" (Insel and Quirion, 2005). This model fails to account for the etiology of mental disorders, and is a very poor guide to treatment. We are often told that we only have to wait for further progress in neuroscience—breakthroughs are constantly promised that are supposedly just around the corner. Unfortunately, no matter how many corners we turn, answers remain out of sight.

Biological reductionism has come to dominate academic psychiatry. A neuroscience model has been strongly supported by the National Institute of Mental Health (NIMH), whose director is Thomas Insel, a researcher best known for his work on oxytocin in prairie voles. Although the media have sometimes described Dr. Insel as America's "psychiatrist-in-chief," this is far from the case. The NIMH director actually favors the abolition of psychiatry, which he thinks should reunite with neurology (Insel and Quirion, 2005). As of 2013, to apply for research grants at NIMH, investigators have been advised to eschew *DSM-5* in favor of a new system, the Research Domain Criteria (RDoC; Insel, 2009; Insel et al., 2010). The RDoC system describes a matrix of dimensions of psychopathology, theoretically evolved and assessed across multiple levels. The data supporting this new system are at best sketchy, and mostly absent. To be confident that the blanks will eventually be filled in, one would have to be a "true believer."

In the meantime, psychiatrists continue to practice their craft and treat very difficult patients. They cannot wait 50 years for a brave new world of neuroscience to come to fruition. We don't know the ultimate fate of systems like the RDoC, but similar proposals have been made in the past (Eisenberg, 1986), and they are now remembered only as historical curiosities.

Fortunately, you don't have to understand clinical phenomena on a molecular or cellular level to make a diagnosis. Psychiatry may not be as precise as other branches of medicine, but by using careful clinical observation, we succeed in helping most of our patients. Moreover, some of the most important empirical findings that have made psychiatry effective were based on observation, rather than on laboratory data. We did not need neuroscience to describe bipolar-I disorder and to determine that it responds specifically to lithium. (Moreover, we still don't know how lithium works in the brain.) In the psychotherapies, where the number of evidence-based treatments has steadily increased, we do not need neuroscience to determine that specific psychological interventions are effective in a wide range of conditions, including depression, anxiety, eating disorders, and personality disorders.

Nonetheless, diagnosis in psychiatry would have a more secure grounding if observation of signs and symptoms could be supplemented by biomarkers. These measures could also turn out to be relevant for disorders with psychosocial determinants, since psychological processes have their own effects on the brain. So why doesn't psychiatry have any biomarkers? A look at the history of medical diagnosis may help shed light on that question.

BIOMARKERS IN MEDICINE AND PSYCHIATRY

Until about a hundred years ago, medical diagnosis was as problematic as psychiatric diagnosis is today. Patients were classified by signs and symptoms such as anemia, swelling, or pain—describing symptoms or syndromes, not diseases with a definite cause or course. Treatment was also symptomatic, and the concept of disease entities only gradually emerged.

In the late nineteenth century, physicians learned how to identify specific etiologies for conditions such as infectious diseases, caused by microorganisms that could be cultured and observed under a microscope. Physicians also learned to validate clinical diagnoses by conducting autopsies and biopsies, allowing for direct observation of pathological changes in organs. These methods proved invaluable in many diseases. Even so, much of medicine remained in a muddle about classifying disease—until technologies were developed to assess markers in living patients. These blood tests and imaging techniques are the backbone of modern diagnosis.

Thus medicine becomes more scientific when biomarkers provide objective measures of disease processes, even if they are not yet available for all diagnoses that physicians treat. (Some conditions remain syndromes, much as in psychiatry.) Biochemical measurements can assess the physiological changes associated with illness. Imaging allows observation of the organs of the body in situ, and can pinpoint abnormalities that previously could only be guessed at. In recent years, a few diseases have also been linked to changes in the genome. All these methods will continue to shape medical diagnosis in the twenty-first century.

Psychiatry has not yet found similar ways to validate its diagnoses, and it entirely lacks biomarkers. In spite of all the progress in neuroscience over the last 20 years, we are still waiting for findings that can be applied to clinical practice.

At this point, there are none (Hyman, 2011). Unfortunately, the hype around neuroscience, with its beautifully colored pictures of brain activity, has deluded many into believing that it has all the answers (Satel and Lilienfeld, 2013). No patient has yet benefited from any of these scientific advances.

Over the years there have been a number of false starts. Blood tests are not helpful in psychiatry: due to the blood-brain barrier, peripheral levels do not necessarily reflect CNS neurochemistry; we can only indirectly measure the activity of neurotransmitters, or of brain hormones. And while these measures are sometimes used in research, they have thus far had no clinical application. Similarly, a large number of studies have applied imaging technologies, usually functional magnetic resonance imaging (fMRI), to mental disorders. But the results are almost always suggestive but nonspecific. While imaging procedures will eventually be refined, they have thus far failed to identify patterns that can be specifically and sensitively correlated with any category of mental illness. Diseases in which a brain lesion can be identified have often become the province of neurology rather than psychiatry. Uher and Rutter (2012) described the impact of neuroimaging on the major mental disorders that psychiatrists treat as essentially "non-informative." There is no way of looking at a brain scan and coming up with any diagnosis.

Genetic studies in medicine have some practical value in oncology, but have been disappointing for psychiatry (Hyman, 2011). None of the genetic markers studied thus far is specific to any diagnosis, and none explains more than 1% of the outcome variance for any disorder. This could be because we don't have the right categories, and have to await the discovery of endophenotypes. Even in disorders in which it is established (from behavior genetics) that heritability is high, we do not know the mechanisms. The main problems derive from complex interactions between multiple genes, from gene-environment interactions, or from epigenetics (the mechanisms determining whether genes are switched on or switched off). This is why expecting to find "genes for" schizophrenia (or any other illness) is naïve (Kendler, 2005). Genetic research could eventually help to identify vulnerabilities, but that development is not likely in the foreseeable future (Uher and Rutter, 2012).

In summary, psychiatry is more or less where the rest of medicine was a hundred years ago—at the very beginning of a long quest for valid diagnostic procedures. This situation should not come as a surprise. If you are studying the liver or the kidney, most cells (or groups of cells) do more or less the same thing. But every neuron in the brain is more or less unique, and there are 100 billion of them, connected in networks that can be counted in the trillions. While research on neural networking might eventually help to sort out this mind-boggling complexity (Zorumski and Rubin, 2011), we are unlikely to find consistent links between psychiatric symptoms and specific regions of the brain. That is because each neural system makes only a small and partial contribution to clinical outcomes. If we do discover biomarkers of this kind, they will probably not look like brain scans, but will reflect a complexity that only some future technology will be able to handle. In summary, the expectation that the kind of breakthrough that created molecular genetics will happen to brain science is attractive to scientists, politicians, and the public at large. But the problem is much too complex for a short-term solution.

Several obstacles interfere with the incremental levels of progress that could be possible in the coming decades. One is that research methods on biomarkers are very expensive, and are often used in small (and inevitably unrepresentative) samples. In neuroimaging, researchers often report differences in samples that rarely exceed 20 subjects. In genetic research, single genes hardly ever have strong effects on their own. One needs very large samples to obtain sufficient power to pick up even the weakest differences, each of which are subject to modulation by other genes, and by the environment.

The story of the search for biomarkers that could validate psychiatric diagnoses is one of short-term frustration but long-term hope. For clinicians, keeping this lack of basic knowledge in mind might help to encourage caution about overdiagnosis.

Finally, biomarkers, even if we were to discover them, would not provide all the data needed to understand how the mind works. Some observers (Fulford et al., 2006) have questioned whether they are either necessary or sufficient to justify a medical diagnosis, and whether relying on them excessively downgrades the psychosocial factors in illness. I would say they are potentially highly useful but conceptually and practically incomplete.

In the past, medicine advanced when new technologies were developed. It could be that yet-to be-developed technologies could change psychiatry within the lifetime of some readers of this book. Even so, it is more realistic to expect incremental change than dramatic breakthroughs. When you are talking about something as complex as the mind, you cannot succeed in reducing thought, emotion, and behavior to cellular mechanisms.

SCREENING AND PSYCHOLOGICAL TESTING

In the absence of biomarkers, psychiatry and clinical psychology have had to focus on *phenomenology*—what can be directly observed by professionals or reported by patients. The art of the clinician lies in asking the right questions, and in observing phenomena accurately. Mental states are measured either by asking patients themselves to describe them, or by having clinicians rate and score them.

These methods can be made more reliable using *psychometrics* (literally, measuring the mind). The most common method in psychology is the use of self-report questionnaires. These instruments are developed using special techniques (item analysis to make sure questions are relevant, and factor analysis to create specific sub-scales). These measures are the backbone of psychological research and have been used to measure everything from personality traits to quality of life. While one might question whether people are always the best judges of their own problems, self-report is usually more reliable than clinical observation.

Since psychologists are interested in normal variation, self-report methods have been widely used in community populations. The question is whether questionnaires are equally useful for clinical diagnosis, or only give the impression of science by providing quantitative scores. In practice, they can only be used as screening measures to identify patients who need to be examined in more detail. As we will see, diagnosing bipolar disorder or attention deficit hyperactivity disorder (ADHD) on the basis of self-report questionnaires has been one of the leading causes of overdiagnosis of these conditions.

The other method of measurement depends on clinical ratings that are scored by practitioners. These "semistructured" interviews present a list of standard questions to guide the rater, who can then ask them in his or her own words. This is the method that underlies *DSM* diagnosis, but formal interviews elaborate the criteria to ensure that nothing important is missed. However, making valid judgments of this kind requires training, since all answers to questions are subject to a degree of interpretation. The advantage of a semi-structured interview is that clinicians cannot skip criteria, or jump to conclusions based on just one of them.

Even so, since there is no "gold standard" for semistructured interviews, and since many are directly based on *DSM* criteria, they can be no more valid than the categories they are designed to measure. These instruments are valuable in research, in that they ensure that patients in a sample have more or less the same psychopathology. But they do not necessarily increase the validity of diagnoses, or prevent overdiagnosis.

One good example is the problems that emerge when similar interviews are used in epidemiological research (Akiskal et al., 2006; Grant et al., 2004). If research assistants, who often administer them, carry out the ratings, the frequency of disorders may not reflect the clinical experience of a better-trained observer. And the most likely problem is not underestimation, but overestimation.

Finally, psychometric data, whether rated by patients or by clinicians, are entirely based on signs and symptoms. They are not necessarily linked to the unknown mechanisms that underlie clinical symptoms, or to biological pathways that could eventually be discovered. No matter how accurate clinical assessment is, diagnostic categories can only be considered provisionally valid, while waiting for a better understanding of mental disorders.

While biomarkers may not provide a complete answer to these questions, they could, at least in principle, be closer to the underlying causes of illnesses. Without them, diagnoses in psychiatry cannot be more than syndromes: convenient ways of communicating about patients with common signs and symptoms. The study of the mind and its maladies remains an enormously complex challenge, full of problems and questions. An honest psychiatrist must accept that answers will require many decades of research. This is where psychiatry is today, and we need to accept these limitations.

OVERDIAGNOSIS AND UNDERDIAGNOSIS

Life is full of decisions that carry potential benefits and risks. These choices can change in the presence of psychopathology. Anxious mood is associated with an overestimation of risk, preventing necessary decisions from being made. Impulsivity produces an underestimation of risk, leading to poorly considered actions that can have negative consequences.

The same dilemmas about risks and benefits apply to clinical assessment. If we underdiagnose patients, we may fail to identify treatable disorders. If we overdiagnose patients, we may treat them for disorders they do not have. Finding the right balance is not easy.

Technically, the consequences of these choices are quantified using the concepts of *sensitivity* and *specificity* (Altman and Bland, 1994). For any disease, there are, at least in principle, true positives, false positives, true negatives, and false negatives. Sensitivity is the proportion of true positives correctly identified, and specificity the proportion of true negatives correctly identified. (The ratio of true positives to true to false positives is the *positive predictive value*.)

Sensitivity and specificity are a trade-off. The right choice depends on whether there is a greater risk in underdiagnosis or in overdiagnosis. When sensitivity is too low, underdiagnosis is likely. But when sensitivity is too high, overdiagnosis is a danger. If you have too many false negatives, you may be missing treatable illness. But when you have too many false positives, your decision-making system has an alarm system that goes off when it shouldn't.

There is a very good reason that overdiagnosis is more likely than underdiagnosis. A bias toward false positives is part of the culture of medicine. Every medical student is taught, above all, not to "miss anything." Yet most conditions that physicians see are, by definition, common. Medicine has an old saw: "when you hear hoofbeats, think horses, not zebras." You can be a good doctor by recognizing the most common clinical presentations, and with experience, it can take only 5 or 10 minutes to identify most of them.

Even so, physicians love to tell stories about missed diagnoses of rare diseases. These incidents often become the subject of clinical-pathological conferences. I remember one from my own student days where the treating physicians failed to recognize an (extremely rare) diagnosis of hyper-parathyroidism. But looking harder for that condition in patients you see in normal practice would be neither practical nor helpful. Fewer medical stories focus on overdiagnoses that lead to useless or harmful treatments. This bias reflects a "can-do" philosophy, in which every effort is made to carry out active interventions, and to search for the diagnostic categories that support doing so.

Psychiatric diagnosis faces a larger hurdle. We can never say that a category is a true positive if we have no "gold standard" on which to base our conclusion. For this reason, specificity and sensitivity often refer to how well observable criteria support a *DSM* diagnosis—which is not the same thing. At best, current diagnoses, based on phenomenology alone, can only be considered to be rough versions of true illnesses that are yet to be discovered.

SCHIZOPHRENIA: OVERDIAGNOSIS AND UNDERDIAGNOSIS

Underdiagnosis is more likely when a disorder is unappealing. That is most likely to happen when the course of the illness is highly chronic, or when effective treatment is complex or inaccessible. A good example is one of the most important conditions in our clinical practice: schizophrenia.

It is difficult to determine whether any mental disorder is underdiagnosed or overdiagnosed. Without a gold standard, one cannot be sure. There are also few empirical studies that can shed light on this issue. But in my professional lifetime I have seen an increasing reluctance on the part of psychiatrists to diagnose schizophrenia.

One might think that a diagnosis so central to psychiatry would not suffer from underdiagnosis. After all, we have powerful tools to manage the psychotic symptoms that mark this illness. But the long-term prognosis of the disorder varies from uncertain to grim. For this reason, psychiatrists may hesitate to diagnose schizophrenia—even when it is obvious.

Yet 50 years ago, American psychiatrists diagnosed *most* psychotic patients with schizophrenia. There was even a category of "pseudo-neurotic schizophrenia" (Hoch et al., 1962), which describes patients who today would be seen as suffering from severe anxiety disorders or personality disorders. The main reason for this diagnosis was the wish to prescribe antipsychotic drugs, which were in their early days of glory, and whose problematic side effects were not yet well known.

Moreover, schizophrenia was too broadly defined 50 years ago, allowing for expansion of the diagnosis. And since lithium was not yet being used, there was little value in differentiating schizophrenia from bipolar disorder. If both types of patients were prescribed antipsychotics, then diagnosis had no effect on treatment. Still another problem was that schizophrenia was (and still is) a heterogeneous syndrome without biological markers; even the course of the disorder is not consistent (Craddock and Owen, 2005).

A research project helped to change the situation. The "New York–London study" (Cooper et al., 1972) showed how fashion in diagnosis can be more important than facts. In the 1960s, researchers interested in differential diagnosis presented filmed interviews of psychotic patients to American psychiatrists (who usually diagnosed them with schizophrenia) and to British psychiatrists (who usually diagnosed them with mania).

In 1970, lithium became widely available. Now differential diagnosis was crucial, since lithium was specific in preventing relapse of manic-depression, which had not been possible when patients were maintained on antipsychotics alone. Then research by Abrams and Taylor (1981) on the differential diagnosis of schizophrenia and bipolar disorder clarified the clinical features of both disorders. It had been widely believed that a set of "first-order" symptoms described by the German psychiatrist Kurt Schneider (1959) were specific to schizophrenia. (That is what I was taught as a resident, and we all dutifully memorized Schneider's list.) But Abrams and Taylor showed that these symptoms are as common in mania as in schizophrenia, and are not specific indicators for either diagnosis.

Younger psychiatrists may not realize that lithium was once a miracle drug—one of the greatest breakthroughs in the history of medical therapeutics. It is understandable that psychiatrists in that era wanted their patients to benefit from it, and were tempted to rediagnose difficult cases as "manic-depressive." Whereas schizophrenia had been overdiagnosed in the past, it now became much less common. Diagnostic fashions can shift from one extreme to another.

Even today, schizophrenia can suffer from under diagnosis. Faced with managing intractable cases, clinicians sometimes look for ways to avoid making this diagnosis. Although some patients show a partial recovery, long-term studies show that its relatively poor prognosis has not changed since the time of Emil Kraepelin, the German psychiatrist who first made the distinction between this type of psychosis and manic-depression (Jobe and Harrow, 2005). This explains a certain preference for diagnoses that focus on mood symptoms.

However, there is also a reason for the reluctance to diagnose schizophrenia to recede. This is due to recent interest in early intervention, with the idea that the disease can be treated more effectively in its early stages (McGorry et al., 2010). However, while identifying schizophrenia in adolescence would have advantages, it has not been shown that early treatment actually improves long-term prognosis.

We have also seen a trend to early diagnosis in other areas of medicine. But this development, however well intentioned, has problems of its own. It is, for example, not clear that everyone with abnormal lipid levels really needs to be on a statin, given that more readily preventable risks, such as hypertension, obesity, smoking, and blood glucose, are the strongest predictors of cardiac disease (Danaei et al., 2009). Practice that focuses more on blood levels than on clinical outcomes reflects a naïve belief in pharmacological intervention that characterizes our medical culture.

Enthusiasm for early treatment of schizophrenia led to a proposal for including a category of "risk psychosis" in *DSM-5* (Addington et al., 2008). This idea was eventually shelved when it became clear that among young people with symptoms that seem to suggest an early onset of schizophrenia, only 30% actually go on to develop psychosis (Bosanac et al., 2010). Thus, including risk psychosis would have led to unnecessary antipsychotic prescriptions in people who do not need them. This example illustrates how the wish to treat, even before a disease develops, can be an important driver of overdiagnosis.

Because of a reluctance to diagnose schizophrenia, as well as the unclear boundary between schizophrenia and bipolarity, a diagnosis of *schizo-affective disorder* is sometimes made, particularly when patients do not have what clinicians believe to be classical symptoms of the disorder (Pope and Lipinski, 1978). But what are the "classical" features of schizophrenia? The image of a chronic patient with limited emotional range ("flat affect") may not be as common as clinicians believe. Schizophrenia patients can become depressed, and about 5% will eventually commit suicide (Palmer et al., 2005).

Schizo-affective disorder is a final twist to the story of the problems that clinicians have in putting patients in valid categories. It is a "fudge" diagnosis, applied to bipolar patients who are more psychotic than clinicians expect them to be. Yet with careful study of clinical features and family history, most patients can be slated either into schizophrenia or bipolar disorder (Lake and Hurwitz, 2006). It is only appealing because it is seen as having a more favorable prognosis.

The reluctance to recognize a serious illness like schizophrenia reflects a universal human tendency to resist bad news. However, psychiatrists cannot make difficult patients go away by failing to diagnose them.

WHY OVERDIAGNOSIS IS THE GREATER PROBLEM

Just as underdiagnosis derives from therapeutic pessimism, overdiagnosis emerges from outbreaks of optimism. Also, the loose use of terms to describe drugs is seriously misleading. Antipsychotics do much more than control psychosis, effects of antidepressants are not specific to depression, and mood stabilizers do not necessarily stabilize mood.

Yet given the enthusiasm about developments in psychopharmacology, after the introduction of antipsychotics, even schizophrenia became a more popular category. At around the same time, as tricylic antidepressants were found to be efficacious, clinicians were attracted by a concept of "masked depression" (Razali, 2000), which suggested that patients without depressive symptoms could respond to antidepressant drugs. Actually, these agents do have a much wider range of indications, and are often effective in anxiety disorders

(Casacalenda and Boulanger, 1998). Pharmacological agents often have broad spectrum effects that go beyond any single category. One cannot conclude from that observation that every clinical picture that responds to an antidepressant is "really" depression.

With the popularity of second-generation antidepressants, primary care physicians became less reluctant to prescribe medication. Patients who respond to serotonin reuptake inhibitors benefited from this development. Unfortunately, a large number of patients do not respond, or have only a placebo response, to these agents (Kirsch et al., 2008). Ironically, optimism about the effects of antidepressants has greatly fueled placebo responses in patients.

In the mental disorders that have vastly increased in prevalence in recent decades, optimism about pharmacological treatment lay behind what proponents call "increased recognition" of a diagnostic category. The first is major depression (Patten, 2008), in which diagnosis has been associated with the wish to prescribe antidepressants. The second is bipolar disorder, now often diagnosed in a broad "spectrum" (Paris, 2012), in which the wish is to prescribe mood stabilizers (and/or antipsychotics). The third is ADHD, driven by a wish to prescribe stimulants (Frances, 2013). In all three cases, optimism has also spread to epidemiological research, and we have seen a dramatic increase in prevalence, both in community studies and in clinical populations. This could represent increased recognition of diagnostic entities, but it could also be a fad for giving patients diagnoses that suggest a specific form of treatment.

Two other conditions have dramatically increased in prevalence for rather different reasons. The first is post-traumatic stress disorder (PTSD), a diagnosis that entered the

DSM manual only in 1980 (McNally, 2003). While there are evidence-based treatments for PTSD, there is no quick fix. Social and political forces, such as the widespread sympathy for victims, not radical optimism about treatment, drive the increased use of this diagnosis. Patients with this condition have always existed, but what has changed is an attribution of their symptoms to the effects of traumatic experiences. In addition, making the diagnosis allows patients to obtain fairly generous disability benefits.

Another diagnosis that has been increasing rapidly in prevalence is autism (and autism spectrum disorders). In this case, there is little reason for therapeutic optimism, since no existing treatment has been found to be more than marginally effective (McPheeters et al., 2011). Yet autism describes a set of serious symptoms for which both families and professionals have sought a diagnostic home. By placing a disparate group of developmental disorders in one category, research is encouraged, and hopes for an eventual cure are raised. Another reason for the popularity of this diagnosis may be the availability of benefits for long-term disability.

ORDER AND CHAOS

The world is full of chaotic events. In psychiatry, since clinical phenomena are complex and difficult to classify, psychiatrists are still searching for a Linnaeus or Mendeleev to put order into chaos. Minds crave meaning, which helps explain the continued influence of traditional religious beliefs, in which unpredictable events reflect supernatural intent. The American psychologist Paul Bloom (2004) has shown that a search for order begins early in infancy, and that young babies behave in ways that are consistent with a concept of cause and effect.

But the human mind's preference for order leads to many incorrect conclusions (Kahnemann, 2011). Connections often follow the principle of "post hoc, ergo propter hoc," that is, events that follow each other in temporal sequence must be causally related. This kind of thinking, so ubiquitous in medicine (consider, for example, the purported links between vaccination and autism), has led us into to many blind alleys.

In the absence of a broad theory of mental illness, psychiatrists should remain cautious about whether their diagnoses reflect reality. We need to make diagnoses to communicate, and common clinical features can sometimes point to a common etiology and/or a pattern of treatment response. But most of the time, diagnoses are just tags we attach to phenomena we do not understand.

It follows that psychiatrists need to overcome their positivistic medical training, and accept that they are doing the best they can under circumstances of relative ignorance. That is not therapeutic nihilism, but a realistic appraisal of what we know and what we don't know. At the present state of knowledge, psychiatry does not need hundreds of diagnoses, only a few of which have well established validity. Overdiagnosis is an attempt to short-circuit a process of scientific discovery that will require many more decades of research.

THE *DSM* AND ITS DISCONTENTS

RESPONSES TO THE PUBLICATION OF *DSM-5*

The fifth edition of the *Diagnostic and Statistical Manual of Mental Disorders* (*DSM-5*) went to press in May 2013. Its publication was well noted in the media; eager for news, many publications put the story on page 1—but got most of the facts wrong. Some reporters referred to the *DSM* as "psychiatry's bible." (The *DSM* is only a tool, and bibles are not revised every 15 years.) Also, the role of key players in the story was greatly exaggerated. Allen Frances was called America's leading psychiatrist, even though he is retired, and only came back in the limelight to criticize *DSM-5*. Thomas Insel, the director of the National Institute of Mental Health, was called America's "psychiatrist-in chief," even though he is a researcher who does not practice, and who has called for the abolition of psychiatry as a medical specialty (Insel and Qurion, 2002). But then the media always love a story.

The publication of *DSM-5* also made waves among practicing psychiatrists. Many were worried that they would have to relearn psychiatry, as many of us in an older generation did in 1980 when the third edition (*DSM-III*) came out. This edition was a truly radical document that created a paradigm shift: diagnosis was made by counting up signs and symptoms, and was not based on unproven theoretical assumptions. *DSM-IV*, published 14 years later, made only minor changes to its predecessor. There is not much of a news story in saying that *DSM-5* is mostly like *DSM-IV*, and that the most radical proposals for the fifth edition were rejected. While *DSM-5* will now become standard, it will not change psychiatry very much.

The media also put the spotlight on the critics of *DSM-5*. Many educated people depend on the *New York Times* to keep up with medicine and science, but newspapers do not review scientific books; rather, they comment on volumes written for the general public.

Two books about *DSM-5* were reviewed in the *New York Times Sunday Book Review* in May 2013. The first was by Gary Greenberg (2013), a psychotherapist who never finished a PhD. Greenberg has previously published critiques of psychiatry, but this book, although uninformed, was savage. It was also gossipy, making it a fun read, even if it had low scientific value. Greenberg has evidently joined the ranks of anti-psychiatrists, since he entirely rejects a medical model for most mental disorders.

The second book was by Allen Frances (2013), who is by far the best informed and the most articulate of the critics of *DSM-5*. Frances, formerly a prominent academic psychiatrist, was the editor of *DSM-IV*. Although the leaders of *DSM-5* were not interested in his opinions, he mounted an effective campaign against the new edition by writing articles in *Psychology Today, Huffington Post*, and *Psychiatric Times*, as well as by writing op-eds in the *New York Times*. Frances's main point was that the new edition threatens an unprecedented expansion of psychiatry into the realm of normality.

He warned that almost every human foible can now be diagnosed as a mental disorder. But the very same point can be made about all previous editions of the *DSM*, including the edition that Frances edited. The reasons for overdiagnosis lie deeper than what is written in any version of the diagnostic manual.

HISTORY OF THE *DSM* SYSTEM

To understand *DSM-5*, we need to go back to the introduction of a new system in 1980. *DSM-III* led to a radical change in the way psychiatry defined itself: the specialty that once claimed to have the key to the human condition converted itself into another branch of medicine. Psychiatrists wanted to be just like other doctors, concentrating on making diagnoses and writing prescriptions. There were, of course, other reasons for a paradigm shift. The authors of *DSM-III* were convinced that they had created a more scientific system of classification. But whatever the original intention, the manual became a tool that supported radical changes in psychiatry, which now focused its energies almost exclusively on psychopharmacology.

The controversy over *DSM-5* was mild by comparison with the intense and emotional arguments about *DSM-III* (Decker, 2013). To put the story in context, psychiatry had been in crisis in the 1960s and 1970s—its very legitimacy was being challenged, and something had to be done. Part of the problem was the dominance in academic circles of an unscientific theory, psychoanalysis. Another part was the inability of psychiatrists to make reliable diagnoses using tools such as *DSM-II*. The American Psychiatric Association, led by its director, Melvin Sabshin, wanted a new system to ensure that psychiatry could be seen as a branch of scientific medicine.

DSM-III, like its successors, did not eliminate the stigma attached to mental disorders (Corrigan, 2005), nor did it silence those who refused to believe that they are real. Attacks on psychiatry do not generally reflect humanistic concern for patients, but the stigma attached to having a disorder. This is inevitable because almost everyone is afraid of mental illness. Some people react by attacking the professionals who treat people who have these disorders. Because of stigma, psychiatry has always had (and always will have) enemies.

DSM-III was a watershed in the history of psychiatry, because by trying to make diagnosis more scientific, it made it important (Decker, 2013). I had been taught *DSM-I* in medical school and *DSM-II* in residency, but these earlier editions were hardly central to practice. In contrast, *DSM-III* was a revolutionary document that required every mental health clinician to follow formal procedures for diagnosis. Developed by Columbia University psychiatrist Robert Spitzer, it replaced descriptive prototypes (which have very low reliability) with algorithms in which diagnoses are made by counting criteria. Even if you don't know the etiology of a disorder, you could still classify it on the basis of signs, symptoms, and course over time. Another revolutionary element was that *DSM-III* was intended to be "atheoretical," avoiding the errors of *DSM-I* and *DSM-II*, many parts of which were based on theories that turned out to be completely wrong.

DSM-III was a key element in psychiatry's paradigm shift. Psychoanalysts, who never liked diagnosis, opposed the new edition because they perceived it (correctly) as an assault on their discipline. The analytic community even threatened to secede from psychiatry. So Spitzer made a compromise: instead of eliminating categories previously grouped under "neurosis" (a concept that psychoanalysts held dear), the term was put in *parentheses* as an alternative. Seven years later, in *DSM-III-R*, "neurosis" was quietly dropped—and nobody missed it.

Psychiatry's paradigm change was necessary, but something important was lost. Although many leaders in the field encouraged the use of a biopsychosocial model (Engel, 1980), practitioners were now tempted to practice in a robotic way, checking *DSM* criteria at each visit. Instead of listening to patients or inquiring about current life circumstances, psychiatrists only monitored the presence of *DSM* criteria. But the system was applied in ways that became a travesty of assessment. In the notorious practice of 15-minute "medication checks," patients complain of symptoms, there is no time to inquire into their causes, but medications intended to remove them tend to be changed frequently. One might argue, however, that this travesty was also supported by a reimbursement system that paid more for seeing three patients for 15 minutes than it did for seeing one for 45 minutes. And because time is of the essence, diagnosis was not made by careful assessment with semi-structured interviews, but by rapid impressions based on *DSM* criteria, or at least the parts of the manual that were easiest to remember.

The *DSM* manual was never intended to support any particular method of treatment. While originally intended to introduce a degree of order into the chaos of psychopathology, it did become a kind of "bible," in the sense that it was wrongly given the prestige of a scientific document. Moreover, the *DSM* system has been linked to a practice in which psychopharmacology is dominant, and in which psychotherapy is no longer practiced. To some extent, psychiatrists are just "following the money." But one also wonders if they have lost interest in what has long made the specialty unique—a profound interest in understanding the human condition.

HOW DIFFERENT IS *DSM*-5?

The short answer is "not much" (Paris, 2013a). There were some radical proposals for *DSM-5* (risk psychosis as a new diagnosis, and a trait-based system for personality disorders), but they were not accepted into the main text of new edition. (Curious readers can find them in "Section III"—a list of conditions requiring further study.) A few changes have opened the door more widely for overdiagnosis, but most problems were already inherent in the system, and are not much worse than in past editions.

DSM-III was criticized for its innovations, but insufficient attention was given to its tendency to support overdiagnosis. Traditional categories became ever more inclusive, while many new categories were introduced. It seemed that almost every kind of psychological problem, even those intrinsic to the human condition, could be described by a psychiatric diagnosis. In part, this reflected the wish of the American Psychiatric Association to validate what many of its members were already doing (i.e., treating normal people with problems). But it also reflected the wish of academic psychiatrists to expand the domain of their concerns. As Frances (2013) pointed out, it is impossible to find experts who think that any of their favorite conditions are being overdiagnosed.

Another issue is that the diagnoses used since *DSM-III* have never been properly researched for reliability and validity. In principle, every category in the manual could have been a subject for investigation, the results of which could have led to empirically based changes in diagnostic criteria. But that is not what happened. Instead, researchers accepted *DSM-III* as if it were a gold standard, and went on to study the relations of its diagnoses to other variables. A good example is epidemiology, which has applied the *DSM* system with unjustified zeal since 1980.

Allen Frances, when he edited *DSM-IV*, made an attempt to curb the excesses of *DSM-III*. Frances took the position that a manual should deliberately avoid making radical changes—unless strongly justified by research—and emphasized that the classification must remain provisional and pragmatic. But some of the changes that worked their way in, albeit with a degree of research support, were a later cause of regret. Twenty years later, Frances, (2013) felt that the wider definitions of bipolarity and adult ADHD that he agreed to had done real damage to patients.

When it came time to prepare *DSM-5*, the editors, David Kupfer of Pittsburgh and Darryl Regier of the American Psychiatric Association, had ambitious goals (Kupfer and Regier, 2011). They hoped to go beyond observable phenomena, and to base diagnosis on biomarkers linked to neuroscience. But since there are no biomarkers in psychiatry, that was not a possibility. The "diagnostic spectra" and "cross-cutting diagnoses" they espoused ended up in Section III of the manual. Kupfer and Regier had hoped for a "paradigm shift" as significant as the one that created *DSM III*. They were hoping for research breakthroughs that would illuminate the endophenotypes that underlie mental illness. They even imagined revising the manual frequently (*DSM 5.1* or *5.2*) each time a breakthrough occurred. At our current stage of knowledge, these were unrealistic dreams, and could only be long-term goals.

DSM-5 also aimed to describe disorders dimensionally and provide a system for quantitative scoring (Kupfer and Regier, 2011). They thought that the proposed "spectra" could have stronger correlations with neurobiological measures. But evidence for the spectra was weak, and biomarkers lack consistent relationships with either categories *or* spectra. DSM-5 had no choice but to continue relying on observable signs and symptoms.

DSM-5 AND THE IDEOLOGY OF CONTEMPORARY PSYCHIATRY

Even before DSM-5 was published, it had generated a large scientific literature. By 2013, 600 published journal articles had already been published. In addition to the popular books on DSM-5, some were written for mental health professionals. I co-edited one of these (Paris and Phillips, 2013); and authored another (Paris, 2013a). Black and Grant (2014) later published a detailed commentary on all the changes in the revised manual. While most books and articles for the general public consisted of criticism, the scientific community examined the pros and cons of specific changes. There was no justification for a broad attack on the manual as a whole.

If you are worried about overdiagnosis in psychiatry, you need to focus on its practitioners, not on its manual. In short, DSM-5 is not the problem, but the way we over-value it is. Making diagnoses gives the impression of hard science at a time when research is in its very early stages. In the absence of solid data, we reify diagnoses that pretend to, but fail to explain mental illness. We can raise or lower diagnostic thresholds, but all that does is to change the frequency of false positives and false negatives (Zimmerman et al., 2010). It does not increase validity—that requires understanding what actually causes mental disorders.

The *DSM* system has pragmatic value as shorthand communication. Its categories are convenient labels, but they should not be thought of as "real" diseases. It may be easier for oldsters like me to understand this point, after living through five editions, none of which was able to answer the most basic questions about psychopathology. But for younger psychiatrists, it is tempting to unconditionally embrace a system that has been around, with only minor changes, for 35 years.

DSM-5, originally billed as a paradigm shift, backed off from radical change. After all the hype and hoopla, the end product was not that different from *DSM-IV* or *DSM-III*. The reason was that when some proposals met a barrage of criticism, the leaders of the American Psychiatric Association became worried. They set up a Scientific Review Committee that was independent of the process of creating the manual to determine whether changes have enough empirical justification. It was headed by two academic luminaries: Kenneth Kendler (editor of *Psychological Medicine* and a leader in behavioral genetic research) and Robert Freedman (editor of the *American Journal of Psychiatry* and a well-known researcher on schizophrenia). Kendler and Freedman adopted the position that no major revisions should be allowed without out strong scientific evidence. And since most of the evidence was weak, few controversial changes were adopted.

While it is good to make it difficult to add disorders to *DSM-5*, applying the same criteria to *removing* disorders from the manual creates other problems. Once a category is included, it is very difficult to take it out without strong scientific evidence. This leads to a manual that is over-crowded with diagnoses that are hardly ever used (Rutter and Uher, 2012). It also keeps categories in the manual that were acceptable in one era, but have long since been discredited by research, such as dissociative disorders (Paris, 2012b).

RESEARCH DOMAIN CRITERIA

Just prior to the publication of *DSM-5*, Thomas Insel, direc-tor of the National Institute of Mental Health (NIMH), made headlines by publicly (and sarcastically) rejecting *DSM-5*. Insel (2009) had already argued that most *DSM* diagnostic categories are invalid because they are not based on neurobi-ology. As a replacement, Insel has developed a set of Research Domain Criteria (RDoC), based on dimensions thought to have neurobiological correlates. In other words, diagnosis would be based not on illness categories, but on a series of scores rated by clinicians.

The RDoC system has been under study by the NIMH (Insel et al., 2010), and workshops have been held to work out a large-scale research program. The RDoC concept fol-lows logically from Insel's belief that mental disorders are brain disorders, and that psychiatry should become a branch of neurology. It is a matrix of theoretical and interlocking dimensions of psychopathology (negative valence, i.e., anxi-ety and depression; positive valence, i.e., reward motivation; cognitive systems; systems for social processes; arousal and regulation systems) across various levels of analysis (genes, molecules, cells, circuits, physiology, behavior, self-reports, and paradigms). At this point, the RDoC system is almost entirely provisional, with most of the boxes either left blank, or partially filled by sketchy findings. Although the NIMH will now require applications for research grants to be framed by RDoC, the system is in a primitive state, with its ultimate future doubtful.

The RDoC system is certainly no better than *DSM-5* in grounding diagnosis in neuroscience. The problem is much the same—everything you can measure is based on symptoms, and nothing is based on endophenotypes.

Kupfer and Regier (2011) stated that while they agreed with Insel in principle, they considered that the data remain insufficient for such a radical change. Why then did Michael First, a researcher from Columbia University and a prominent figure in the development of *DSM-IV*, become a supporter, describing RDoC as "the future of diagnosis" (First, 2011)? While I don't know the answer, to adopt a system that has even *less* research behind it than the current manual is hardly progressive. Moreover, the RDoC system is *not* based on neuroscience (unless one counts theories on the same level as empirical findings).

This story will probably be one more broken promise from the neuroscience community, which has too often claimed that a biological understanding of mental illness is imminent, and then has failed to deliver the goods. Finally, like all dimensional systems, the RDoC system assumes that there is no boundary between psychopathology and normality. If the future has indeed arrived, it will encourage clinicians to diagnose mental disorders in just about anyone.

DIMENSIONAL DIAGNOSIS

The *DSM-5* vision to *dimensionalize* diagnosis would have required clinicians to make quantitative scores of pathology. There is a major disconnect between clinicians who use categories to make treatment decisions, and researchers who believe that quantitative scoring of traits or symptoms is a better way to illuminate fundamental mechanisms. Yet by rejecting the approach of *DSM-III*, in which mental disorders were seen as distinct entities, psychiatry seems, rather ironically, to be returning to the heyday of psychoanalysis, claiming that all psychopathology lies on a continuum with normality.

In principle, one could dimensionalize any aspect of psychopathology. We already do so with rating instruments like the Hamilton scales for depression (HAM-D) and for anxiety (HAM-A), as well as the Global Clinical Impression for symptoms of all kinds. These scores provide quantitative additions to qualitative judgments required to make categorical diagnosis. They are useful for determining severity, but this is not the same as using dimensions to replace categories.

Proposals for the classification of personality disorder (PD) in *DSM-5* were intended as a "poster child" for the eventual dimensionalization of all diagnoses in the manual. Many experts in trait psychology (Costa and Widiger, 2013) had called for dimensions to replace categories. Yet while the PD work group for *DSM-5* spent five years on its proposal, it only produced disagreement and failure (Gunderson, 2013).

This story has lessons for the future of diagnosis, as well as for overdiagnosis. The PD proposal would have kept some of the categories, but would base them on ratings of trait dimensions, to be scored by clinicians. The problem would have been that, without extensive training, these ratings would have been unreliable. Moreover, a "hybrid" system of categories and dimensions turned out to be complex and unwieldy, sorely lacking in clinical utility. Even if it had been adopted, it would probably have never been used.

The Scientific Committee rejected the hybrid proposal and consigned it to Section III, and the *DSM-IV* criteria were retained word for word. The moral of the story is that it is better to keep a bad system that everyone is familiar with, than to institute radical changes without strong scientific evidence. Moreover, for conditions like PDs that are usually underdiagnosed (Zimmerman et al., 2010), it hardly made sense to make it even more difficult to identify them.

LESSONS FROM THE STORY OF *DSM-5*

Changes in the *DSM*, even small ones, can run the risk of creating more diagnostic epidemics. But psychiatry has already had its share of epidemics, and most of them occurred under *DSM-III* and *DSM-IV*.

DSM-5 can be no more and no less valid than the current state of psychiatry. Overdiagnosis is not a direct consequence of what is written in this manual. Everything depends on how the system is used. Most problems come from the wish of clinicians to identify conditions they believe they can treat. These difficulties do not lie with any particular edition, or with the wording of any particular set of criteria. Zimmerman and Galione (2010) showed that *DSM* is not followed, even when diagnosing major depression. Clinicians have never followed the manual very carefully, and probably never will.

This having been said, we can draw a few lessons from the story of *DSM-5*. The first is that you can't create a scientific manual out of nothing. If we don't have the data, we should make do with what we have, and wait for further research.

The second is that the leaders of the *DSM-5* Task Force, and of the work groups that reviewed criteria for specific disorders, were full-time academics who do not work in the trenches, and who only manage a small number of treatment-resistant cases. Experts who write a manual that is used by every mental health professional need to keep their fingers on the clinical pulse.

The third is that the *DSM-5* was not properly tested, particularly for reliability. The field trials conducted in 2011 were begun after the manual was essentially written, so they did not lead to any changes. Moreover, the reliability of some of the most basic diagnoses in psychiatry was surprisingly poor. Regier et al. (2013) reported that confidence intervals at multiple sites had little overlap, and that pooled results were acceptable at only one of two sites. While the authors claimed "good" test-retest reliability for bipolar I disorder, borderline personality disorder, schizoaffective disorder, alcohol use disorder, and binge eating disorder, all were supported by only one acceptable trial, and were not replicated at a second site. Only three adult diagnoses (PTSD, complex somatic symptom disorder, and major neurocognitive disorder) obtained an intra-class kappa in the good or very good range at multiple sites. Moreover, reliability would probably have been even lower in ordinary clinics that did not have access to experts.

Positive conclusions about low levels of reliability in *DSM-5* are based on the assumption that it is no worse in psychiatry than in other medical specialties (Kraemer et al., 2012), as well as the fact that many cases have heavy comorbidity, which makes it difficult to determine which diagnosis is most important. But the suggestion of Kraemer et al. (2012), on behalf of the *DSM-5* leadership, that kappas as low as .20 can be considered "acceptable" was something of a shocker. While some new diagnoses that were proposed, such as a proposal for mixed anxiety and depression, were shelved because of unreliability, several of the most familiar categories did so poorly in the field trials that one has to wonder why major depression didn't meet the same fate.

It would be good if psychiatry had made a little more progress in making more reliable diagnoses in the last few decades. But the most important lesson is not to take the categories in current use too seriously.

HOW THE *DSM* SYSTEM IS USED TO JUSTIFY OVERDIAGNOSIS

DSM-III, and all its revisions, had a note in its introduction specifically stating that a diagnostic manual was not intended as a guide to treatment. Yet that is how the manual has often been used. Diagnosing mental disorders, instead of requiring training and experience, has become a game any physician can play—all you have to do is count the criteria and write a prescription. (Even patients can follow the same process by looking up their diagnosis on the Web.) A mindless application of the *DSM* to clinical practice has produced a generation of psychiatrists who can be as insensitive as any internist. The *DSM* is used to justify overdiagnosis in psychiatry, mainly because physicians are afraid of "missing something." And how do you know whether you are missing anything if you haven't asked all the questions?

More practically, *DSM* criteria can guide our questions when diagnosis is unclear. But nothing in the manual forces us to interview patients in a way that focuses *only* on whether they meet a set of criteria for a specific category. For example, it is not necessary, even in the absence of grounds for a clinical suspicion of bipolarity, to run through a long series of questions about mania and hypomania. That should only be done when there are good reasons to suspect the presence of a bipolar disorder.

Every question in a diagnostic interview takes time from another potential question. You need to cover symptoms as well as a life history, and you usually have less than an hour to do so. If you spend too much time on *DSM* criteria, you won't get to explore the impact of life events. The manual doesn't force you to conduct interviews robotically. Yet sometimes tools take over the people who use them.

3

OVERDIAGNOSIS AND
OVER-TREATMENT

WHY PSYCHIATRY EMBRACED OVERDIAGNOSIS

Overdiagnosis is driven by optimism about treatment methods, while underdiagnosis is driven by pessimism about treatability. Neither practice reflects the purpose of diagnosis in medicine. Classifying disease is a way of understanding it, and does not necessarily lead to conclusions about therapy. For example, important research has been conducted for decades on multiple sclerosis, and the cause of this terrible disease will eventually be found. Yet the progress that has been made has had little effect on our ability to help patients who have that diagnosis.

Thus scientific knowledge should be the driving force behind diagnostic classification. Each category of illness must be a meaningful entity with a specific etiology and a specific pathogenesis. Instead of shoe-horning patients into diagnoses for which we already have treatments, we need to carry out more research on conditions for which we don't have effective therapy. In the long run, a valid diagnosis provides a target for empirical investigations to uncover causes, and then to lead the way to better treatment. But the first step is to be honest about our ignorance.

Psychiatrists find it hard to accept that they still lack a basic understanding of most forms of mental illness. Yet paradoxically, this very lack of knowledge about the causes of disorders is what makes overdiagnosis attractive. Putting a patient in a well-known category gives the impression of science and justifies using whatever tools clinicians already have.

For the last hundred years, psychiatrists have wanted to make the same progress that has marked the history of internal medicine. The first step could be an empirically supported classification. The leader of the movement to make diagnosis scientific was the German psychiatrist Emil Kraepelin. Realizing that too little was known about the brain to account for mental disorders, Kraepelin (1921) created a system defined by symptoms, course, and prognosis. Illnesses with specific patterns could represent unique entities. It was left to later generations to fill in the blanks by discovering the neural mechanisms behind psychopathology. But that was a hundred years ago, and we are still more or less in the same position.

Many of Kraepelin's ideas continue to be influential in the twenty-first century. Psychiatry later renamed dementia praecox "schizophrenia," and manic-depression "bipolar disorder," but the distinction between these two conditions, based on a difference between worsening chronicity and episodic illness, remains seminal. In spite of significant overlap between these diagnoses (Craddock, 2005), many lines of research have vindicated Kraepelin's approach. Most important, bipolar disorder responds to lithium, while schizophrenia does not.

The rise of "neo-Kraepelinian" psychiatry (Klerman, 1986) was an attempt to return to an older model, associated with a rejection of Freud (who was not interested in diagnosis). The aim was to discover categories of illness for which specific treatments could be developed. At the time, these ideas were revolutionary, because they overthrew a "one size fits all" approach that had made diagnosis seem irrelevant.

Psychoanalysis became prominent in American psychiatry because it filled a niche and was an attractive antidote to therapeutic nihilism (Paris, 2005). Sixty years ago, no effective biological treatment, other than electroconvulsive therapy, was available (Shorter, 1997). Psychoanalysis claimed to be a complete theory of the mind, and a comprehensive treatment for every kind of mental illness. But eventually, a fragile evidence base led to its decline. Its theoretical ideas were contradicted by research, and its time-intensive and expensive methods were never subjected to systematic clinical trials. This is why other physicians rightly viewed us with suspicion, and why psychiatrists eventually rejected the model, replacing it with a neo-Kraepelinian perspective that had a strong resemblance to internal medicine.

This story may not seem of interest to younger clinicians, but it is instructive. Physicians are more interested in practice than in theory. When a model fails to deliver the goods of effective treatment, it gets dropped. The same thing may be happening now to the neo-Kraepelinian model, which, with the important exception of lithium therapy, has not led to great breakthroughs in treatment. Newer models, based on fashionable trends in neuroscience, have become the focus of hope.

The greatest breakthroughs in psychiatric treatment occurred decades ago. Since the introduction of lithium in

1970, our pharmacological armamentarium is no better than it was then, even if side effect profiles are more favorable. The 1950s and 1960s were the glory days of the psychopharmacological revolution, and I am old enough to have lived through this "age of miracles." As an undergraduate, I saw what mental hospitals were like before psychiatrists learned how to prescribe antipsychotic drugs. As a psychiatric resident, I was the first physician at my hospital to prescribe lithium to a bipolar patient.

If drugs could cure (or at least control) severe mental illness, then practitioners were bound to see the future of psychiatry as lying in neuroscience. Thus a new generation of psychiatrists aimed to replicate the success of internal medicine, and to identify specific categories of disease that would respond to specific treatments. Unfortunately, this approach was at best a partial success, and at worst a disappointment. With the exception of lithium, the drugs used in psychiatry have broad effects that are not specific to any diagnosis.

The ideas behind *DSM-5* involve a jettisoning of a neo-Kraepelinian approach, replacing it with spectra that would be dimensional rather than categorical (Kupfer and Regier, 2011). A similar point of view lies behind the radical vision of Research Domain Criteria (RDoC; Insel, 2009). These systems would like to replace illness categories with constructs that (hopefully) correspond to neurobiological processes. This is a kind of bet—that when we know more about brain chemistry and connectivity, a new and more powerful theory about the causes of mental illness will emerge. The bet could well be lost.

No one can doubt the enormous progress that has been made in neuroscience in the last few decades. When

I compare our current level of knowledge to what I was taught as an undergraduate, the contrast is dramatic. Yet we still do not know enough to base psychiatric diagnosis on what has been learned about the brain. Few of the advances in neuroscience shed light on specific mental disorders, and this line of research has had little influence on clinical practice (Hyman, 2007). We are promised that breakthroughs are imminent. But the complexity of brain connectivity and functioning makes it doubtful that answers to key questions about mental illness will emerge during the lifetime of any reader of this book.

For now, classification continues to depend not on mechanisms, but on signs and symptoms. That is why *DSM-5* was not radically revised. That is also why all the *DSM* manuals since 1980 have spoken only of "disorders" (carefully avoiding the term *disease*). In reality, the categories we use are not diseases, but *syndromes*. They can be clinically useful for some purposes, but need eventually to be formulated as illnesses with well-understood endophenotypes.

Why do so many psychiatrists see the emphasis on neuroscience as the basis of their practice? The reason is not that neuroscience guides clinical practice—we don't even know how our drugs work in the brain. More important is our image as specialists—we crave the respect of our colleagues and our patients. We want to be scientific practitioners, and to be seen as a medical specialty like any other. That helps explain why *DSM-III* was treated not as a provisional tool, which is all it really ever was, but as a scientific document. But when mental health professionals believe too much in the reality of disorders, they may prescribe treatments that are as doubtful as the diagnoses they are making.

DRUGS AND OVERDIAGNOSIS

When effective treatments appear in medicine, physicians are tempted to give them to more patients. One need only think of the over-prescription of antibiotics for infections of all kinds (including viral diseases that do not respond to these agents). That is what happened when psychiatry finally developed effective drugs for psychoses and severe depression. Antidepressants moved beyond the realm of severe mood disorders, and began to be prescribed to every unhappy person. The most recent data (Pratt et al., 2011) shows that 11% of the adolescent and adult US population is taking one of these agents. The numbers are even higher for women, and show regional variation, with higher rates in large cities.

The expansion of antidepressant prescriptions did not occur immediately after the first effective agents were introduced in the 1950s. This trend was limited for many years due to the unpopularity of tricyclics, which had too many side effects for the average family doctor to manage. But it sped up rapidly when second-generation antidepressants, selective serotonin reuptake inhibitors (SSRIs), which have much more tolerable side effect profiles, became available.

Moreover, studies showing a high frequency of relapse when these drugs were withdrawn (Hansen et al., 2008) encouraged physicians to prescribe antidepressants indefinitely. When I see people who have been on them for decades and will probably never get off, I don't get upset, because their long-term side effects are not usually severe. The one question that comes up with some frequency is whether to stop these agents during a pregnancy.

Antipsychotics are another story. Although they were long used as adjunctive agents in mood disorders, the side effects of "typical" drugs discouraged writing too many prescriptions. But with the arrival of "atypicals," supported by enormous publicity from Big Pharma, they began to move out of their traditional niche: the treatment of psychotic symptoms. One of the most common indications today is the treatment of insomnia (Comer et al., 2011). A combination of antidepressants and antipsychotics for depressed patients, or even the use of atypicals as first-line agents, has also become common.

The hammers of psychopharmacology are now being used for all kind of nails. Lithium and other mood stabilizers are no longer limited to patients with bipolar disorder, but are given to patients who feel moody, and are considered to lie within the "bipolar spectrum" (Paris, 2012). Almost anyone who has trouble with focus and attention can be diagnosed with attention deficit hyperactivity disorder (ADHD) and offered a stimulant (Batstra and Frances, 2012).

To justify the expansive use of psychopharmacology, patients must be diagnosed with conditions that are indications for any of these treatments. Otherwise, most of psychiatry would have to be practiced "off-label." (This has already happened, but overdiagnosis masks the trend.) The wish to prescribe has turned into a wish to find more diagnoses in more patients.

This trend has been supported by the pharmaceutical industry, which wants *everyone* to take drugs. They advertise their products directly to consumers, who are gently advised to "ask their doctor" before trying them. The trend toward overdiagnosis has also been supported by physicians who want to help patients with any sort of problem—and who also want to make more money.

How much does diagnosis really tell you about patients? The answer is—not as much as you think. The most important exceptions are bipolar disorder and schizophrenia. Missing a diagnosis of bipolar-I would deny patients a highly effective drug: lithium. (This inexpensive agent, when properly used, remains the best treatment for the disorder.) Missing schizophrenia would deny these patients the benefit of antipsychotics. These are clinical situations in which diagnosis is not an academic exercise, but leads to life-and-death decisions.

Yet hardly any other category in the manual responds to treatment that is specific to any diagnosis. This conclusion is supported by the fact that antidepressants have effects on anxiety, and by the fact that both antidepressants and antipsychotics are highly sedating, putting a cap on whatever symptoms patients suffer from. But while these drugs have broad effects that go beyond any diagnostic category, nobody has shown that they can treat unhappiness.

HOW EPIDEMIOLOGY FELL VICTIM TO OVERDIAGNOSIS

Before the age of *DSM-III*, a few intrepid researchers attempted to determine the extent to which mental disorder exists in the community. In the 1950s and early 1960s, pioneering research, such as the Stirling County Study in Canada (Leighton, 1959) and the Midtown Manhattan Study in the United States (Srole and Fischer, 1980), was carried out. These surveys, much like later epidemiological research, reported a surprisingly high level of psychological distress in the community. I can remember from my student days the incredulous response of the media to the Midtown Manhattan Study, which reported that half of the population had significant psychological symptoms. But in the era of *DSM-I*, epidemiologists did not use formal diagnoses to measure psychopathology. Instead, they simply scored people on scales to determine to what extent they were functional or dysfunctional.

When the *DSM-III* system was adopted, epidemiologists began to use it as a primary tool. The Epidemiological Catchment Area (ECA; Robins and Regier, 1991) study of the 1970s and 1980s was the largest survey of mental disorder up to that point, and it was based on categories listed in *DSM-III*. The tradition was carried on by later large-scale surveys based on later editions of the manual: the National Comorbidity Survey (NCS; Kessler et al., 1997) and the National Comorbidity Survey Replication (NCS-R; Kessler et al., 2005).

Nobody stopped to ask how measurements in community samples can be precise when the "gold standard" consists of diagnoses with problematic validity. Few took notice of the circular reasoning in which broad definitions of disorders lead to high levels of prevalence. When the NCS-R reported that a large percentage of the population suffered from depression, bipolarity, ADHD, or autism, one could only argue with the results by questioning the *DSM* system itself. And that is just what should have been done. Instead, epidemiology was used to validate conditions that lacked external validity. For this reason, Allen Frances once told me that epidemiology has done more damage to psychiatry than almost anything else.

The most recent of these studies is the National Epidemiological Study of Alcohol and Related Conditions (NESARC; Grant et al., 2004a). But it was based on *DSM* criteria rated by research assistants, so its findings about personality disorders (PDs) were particularly unbelievable and misleading (Grant et al., 2004b). As an expert on these conditions, I might be biased in favor of diagnosing them. But I refuse to accept that 15%–20% of the population suffer from PDs. That level of extension into normality would make the whole concept meaningless.

People tend to forget that *DSM*, in its various editions, is a method of communication, not a scientifically valid document. The manual was written to allow physicians to justify seeing all kinds of patients. For this reason, many diagnoses have been expanded to meet the needs of practitioners to treat a wide range of patients.

The term *inflated prevalence* refers to the tendency of epidemiological research to over-estimate the frequency of mental disorders in the community (Patten, 2008). Over time, major surveys seem to find more and more people who meet criteria for one or another diagnosis. Prevalence has greatly increased for major depression, bipolar spectrum disorders, ADHD, and autism (Frances, 2013). The main exception is schizophrenia, which has remained at less than 1% in almost all samples (Kessler et al., 2007)— possibly because this is not a condition that epidemiologists are particularly eager to find. Later chapters will examine the causes of inflated prevalence in each of the conditions that have been subject to what might be called diagnostic epidemics.

DIAGNOSTIC EPIDEMICS
IN CLINICAL PRACTICE

Inflated prevalence is by no means confined to epidemiological research, but it has had a profound effect on clinical practice. I am indebted to Allen Frances (2013) for introducing the term *diagnostic epidemic*, which occurs when practitioners see a category in more and more of their patients, leading to rapid increases in clinical prevalence. Epidemics occur even more easily if one accepts simpleminded algorithims. Again, major depression is the best example. If patients are unhappy enough for two weeks or more to have five clinical symptoms, they will meet criteria for the diagnosis. This explains why the diagnosis is so ubiquitous. Epidemics can also happen when patients present with symptoms that superficially resemble an established diagnosis. For example, moodiness can be seen as a form of bipolar disorder. Troubles with attention may be seen as ADHD. People who are strange or nerdy may be diagnosed as autistic. Patients who have had something bad happened to them (either recently or in the past) may receive a diagnosis of post-traumatic stress disorder (PTSD).

One of the quirks of diagnostic epidemics is that they claim to be based on the latest science. Tough questions may not be asked when a diagnostic construct seems to explain so much. And patients readily buy into these ideas. Many announce to their physicians (and their families), "I have been *diagnosed* with...." Patients who talk like this evidently believe they have just undergone a definitive test like a biopsy or a scan. At best, they have been given a self-report measure as a screening tool. And all too often, diagnosis in psychiatry is just one clinician's opinion.

The bandwagon effect of diagnostic epidemics makes physicians vulnerable to what has been called an "availability bias" (Kahnemann, 2011). In other words, they diagnose patients according to what is already on their mind, rather than what they are actually observing.

Still another problem is that clinicians do not always remember what is in the manual, or consult it before coming to a conclusion, as has been clearly shown in empirical research (Zimmerman and Galione, 2010). The process of diagnosis in psychiatry remains "rough and ready," and we cannot expect practitioners to make diagnoses in the precise way recommended by a scientific manual.

DIAGNOSIS, NEUROSCIENCE, AND THE PHARMACEUTICAL INDUSTRY

No discussion of overdiagnosis can be complete without considering the role of the pharmaceutical industry. The worldview of biological psychiatry, in which mental disorders are redefined as brain disorders and are treated with drugs, has been greatly supported by pharmaceutical companies, which make enormous profits from products that are marketed to billions of people.

At the same time, the pharmaceutical industry pays experts from academia to influence clinicians to prescribe their drugs (Angell, 2000). But why do practitioners accept the message that pharmacology should dominate their therapeutic armamentarium? To understand this phenomenon, we need to consider ideological factors. Again, prescribing drugs makes psychiatry look like the rest of medicine. The view that psychotherapy is at best inefficient, and at worst unscientific, is based on the assumption that mental illness is, in the common parlance, the result of "chemical imbalances" that can be corrected by the right drug cocktail. In this way, the appeal of pharmacology reflects the dominance of a neuroscience model of mental illness. While lip service may be paid to the effects of life experience on psychopathology, many psychiatrists believe that their patients are suffering from problems in neurotransmission and neuroconnectivity. And these ideas make it all too easy to diagnose everyone with some form of mental disorder.

SCIENCE, PHILOSOPHY,

AND DIAGNOSIS

SCIENTIFIC DIAGNOSIS

The empirical study of diagnosis in medicine, or *nosology*, aims to ground categories of illness in scientific data. To accomplish this, researchers determine the *construct validity* of diagnoses—that is, whether they measure what they set out to measure. Studies of construct validity are a basic concept in psychology (Cronbach and Meehl, 1951). Most of the data comes from self-report questionnaires. But since clinical ratings and diagnoses are subjective, they require *external validity*. This means that assessments made by practitioners need to correspond to some other measurement, sometimes called a "gold standard."

In internal medicine, one can compare clinical diagnoses to the results of blood tests, imaging, biopsies, or autopsies. Biomarkers can be open to interpretation—for example, radiologists may not always agree about the results of a scan. But when biomarkers are specific and sensitive, they do illuminate disease processes. Psychiatry lacks a gold standard, but that may not always remain the case.

In the absence of external validity, signs and symptoms, even though they are inevitably subjective, must be our starting point. What we observe and what patients tell us, as well as the clinical judgments derived from this information, may or may not be reliable.

Research on construct validity in psychiatric diagnosis began more than 40 years ago, when Eli Robins and Samuel Guze (1970), researchers at Washington University in St. Louis, Missouri, developed principles that became the conceptual basis of *DSM-III*. The Robins-Guze criteria for validity were (1) clinical description, (2) laboratory study, (3) exclusion of other disorders, (4) follow-up data, and (5) family history.

Unfortunately, each of these criteria suffers from serious problems (Kendler, 1990). Clinical description is limited by subjectivity and bias: even with systematic training, practitioners have a tendency to see what they expect to see. Laboratory studies of mental illness remain in their infancy, with biomarkers still only a hope for the future. Overlap between diagnoses is common, and zones of rarity between disorders are hardly ever found. Follow-up data are limited by the heterogeneous course of mental illnesses. Finally, while disorders run in families, the most consistent patterns are for symptoms and traits, not for diagnoses. In summary, the Robins-Guze criteria were a noble idea, but they have been a failure in practice, and have not helped psychiatrists to develop a scientific nosology.

Robert Spitzer (1976), the editor of *DSM-III*, developed an alternative approach to construct validity, which he called Longitudinal Evaluation of All Data, or the "LEAD" standard. This simply means that diagnostic conclusions are based on as much information as one can practically gather. But what

LEAD offers is a more formal version of expert consensus, not external validity.

The ultimate source of construct validity in diagnosis could be biomarkers. Without them, one cannot be sure of the validity of the most common diagnoses in psychiatry. Are schizophrenia and bipolar disorder separate diseases or overlapping syndromes? We cannot know—since what defines these conditions are not unique neurobiological processes, but a list of signs and symptoms. Is depression a single disease that varies only in severity? As long as biomarkers are unknown, it is not possible to determine whether that idea is true or false. Does every person who meets the current criteria for ADHD have the same illness? Again, without biomarkers, it is impossible to answer that important question.

The largest and most impressive empirical studies of diagnosis have been conducted by Mark Zimmerman, a psychiatrist trained in Iowa and working at Brown University. Zimmerman's research examines the validity and consistency of clinical assessments in outpatient clinics. Zimmerman's Methods to Improve Diagnostic Assessment and Services (MIDAS) project has thus far produced over 200 scientific papers. (This clinically important project has been carried out without any external funding.)

Strikingly, MIDAS showed that clinicians do not follow the DSM very closely, even for major depression (Zimmerman and Galione, 2010). The reason that diagnosis in practice ignores many of the criteria listed and described in the manual is that practitioners cannot remember them. It has long been known in psychology that any list that has more than seven items will not stay in memory (Miller, 1956). Most people would have trouble listing the Ten Commandments!

Nine criteria for depression are just too many—unless you look them up.

Moreover, when assessments must be made in a few minutes, clinicians are particularly likely not to follow an algorithim. Fast thinking, as Kahneman (2011) has shown, is subject to availability biases, in which the first thing that comes to mind can take precedence. This may explain why, as Zimmerman et al. (2005) found, even if systematic semi-structured interviews are the gold standard, clinical diagnoses in practice are highly inaccurate, over-identifying some of the most popular categories, and missing others.

In short, one cannot apply a scientific nosology to clinical settings if practitioners do not pay careful attention to what is written in the manual. In any case, even the most scrupulous use of *DSM* criteria cannot achieve construct validity until mental disorders are better understood. For psychiatry, validity still remains a long-term goal.

DIAGNOSES AS HEURISTICS

Even if diagnoses are not always scientific, can they still be useful? The answer is yes, because they can serve as *heuristics*. This term refers to rules of thumb based on practical experience, as opposed to theoretically coherent constructs like elements in chemistry or cells in biology. Heuristics differ from scientific methods in being approximate rather than precise. We tend to forget this. When I communicate diagnoses to my colleagues, I know they are not real—but I am not sure that other people understand the principle.

Kahnemann (2011) described the concept of heuristics in some detail. When people lack complete data, as they almost always do (and as clinicians do when making diagnoses), they must rely on rules of thumb. These shortcuts guide us to conclusions that may not be rooted in research, but that provide an efficient way of communicating information.

Heuristics are not "real," but over time, they tend to become *reified*. (This term refers to a process in which an abstraction is treated as if it has concrete existence.) Many diagnoses become popular when they make sense to clinicians. Others have been in the manual for so long that they are no longer questioned.

Major depression is, once again, a prime example. This diagnosis is a heuristic that can sometimes provide practical guidance, but it does not describe a disease process. Rather, major depression is a convenient way of describing a set of clinical phenomena with common features. In other words, it is a syndrome. That is why patients with this diagnosis have such a variable response to treatment. If practitioners considered diagnosis as heuristic, they might not overdiagnose depression, and they might not put every patient who meets diagnostic criteria on an antidepressant. Doing so would implicitly acknowledge that the diagnosis is a heuristic, not a specific entity requiring specific treatment. Unfortunately, that approach, central to medicine, retains its hold on the imagination.

REDUCTIONISM

Reductionism is one of the most successful strategies in science. It is an approach in which complex phenomena are understood by breaking them up into simpler components. Examples include nuclear physics (atoms are made up of quarks and electrons), chemistry (molecules are made up of elements), and biology (organs are made up of cells). In medicine, physicians sometimes speak of "treating the whole person," but usually understand disease at the level of organs, tissues, and cells. It seems natural to assume that the mind, as a function of the brain, can be understood by studying the chemistry and connectivity of neurons. The idea that mental disorders are brain disorders is a strongly held belief among biological researchers in psychiatry (Insel and Qurion, 2002).

The main problem with reductionism is that the world studied by scientific research consists of different levels, each of which needs to be examined in its own right (Gold, 2009; Kirmayer and Gold, 2012). Thus while quarks are an essential concept in nuclear physics, they have little relevance for engineering. In chemistry, molecules (such as water) cannot usually be explained by the nature of the atoms that comprise them. In biology, you cannot fully explain the behavior of organisms by the functioning of their cells. Similarly, in psychiatry, while neural chemistry and connectivity help to explain some phenomena, complex mental states cannot routinely be reduced to a neural level.

Some psychiatrists, particularly those working in academia, are committed to biological reductionism. Many espouse determinism, and consider free will to be an illusion. (If you believe that, it is almost guaranteed that your practice will be restricted to pharmacological interventions.) When I try to explain the limits of reductionism in psychiatry, the suspicion arises that I am a dualist: that I think that the mind has an independent existence from brain. Needless to say, that is not what I believe. I am a materialist, and I know that the mind is entirely a product of neural activity. The point that reductionists miss is that each level of analysis describes characteristics that cannot be explained by reductive procedures. In philosophy these are called *emergent* properties (Gold, 2009). Put simply, the whole is greater than its parts.

The application of purely biological models has done great harm to psychiatry, downgrading the importance of psychosocial factors (Bracken et al., 2012). If you want to understand mental illness, the answer does not necessarily come from monoamine levels or fMRI activity of brain regions. These are clues to the nature of disorders, but they do not provide a full explanation. We need to return to a biopsychosocial model.

Even as neuroscience sheds light on how the brain works, it is unrealistic to expect that the mind will ever be fully explained at the level of neurons. It is a large leap from neural connections and neurotransmitters to the complexities of cognition, emotion, and behavior. When one is considering trillions of potential interactions, as is the case for the brain, reductionism can only be one of several strategies. Ideally, science makes the best progress by analyzing phenomena on multiple levels. Astronomers who study the evolution and structure of galaxies do not explain these phenomena at the level of individual stars. Biologists who study evolution have shown that natural selection, while driven by changes in DNA, only occurs when an organism interacts with its environment.

WHEN DOES MENTAL DISORDER FADE INTO NORMALITY?

The phenomena associated with the diagnosis of any mental disorder could be mapped as a Bell curve. At the peak of the curve are cases so typical that they are uncontroversial. But as one moves to the periphery, patients may suffer from only a few symptoms of a disorder, and may not even experience themselves as ill. This is the uncertain boundary between subclinical and normal. There is no way of drawing a line between them—except arbitrarily, much as we diagnose intellectual deficiency when IQ scores fall more than two standard deviations from a mean.

Thus there has never been a satisfactory definition of a mental disorder. Wakefield (2012) has taken the best shot at it, proposing that disorders are based on the concept of *harmful dysfunction.* By this Wakefield means that a disorder must create significant harm to the individual, and must interfere with functions that are evolutionarily programmed. Even so, it is normal to experience symptoms, and to be dysfunctional in one way or another. At some point you have to make an arbitrary judgment as to whether problems are harmful enough and cause enough dysfunction to justify making a diagnosis.

Normality is an abstraction: a state in which psychopathology is entirely absent. Needless to say, there is no such thing, even in the happiest and most functional people. We all suffer from distress, and almost everyone feels unhappy from time to time. Yet clinicians may be tempted to diagnose these phenomena as subclinical manifestations of illness.

Frances (2013) argues that psychiatry, with support from *DSM-5*, has lost sight of what is normal. The classification system is on its way to diagnosing everyone with some disorder or another. Epidemiological studies based on *DSM* criteria have already shown that most people meet criteria for a mental disorder during their lifetime (Moffitt et al., 2009). Perhaps that is to be expected—after all, the lifetime rate of physical illness is 100%. But lumping normal reactions to circumstance with serious illness trivializes the concept of a disorder. It is true that in medicine the common cold is considered as much an illness as pneumonia. But everyone knows that there is little point in consulting a physician for a cold. The problem with considering reactions to life's vicissitudes as indicators of pathology is that people will be encouraged to seek out treatments, most particularly psychopharmacological treatments, that could be harmful.

Each disease has its advocates, and many experts consider the disorders that interest them to be underdiagnosed. The first paragraph of every research grant application begins with a statement that the disorder under study has a high prevalence. Nobody wants to spend money on rare diseases.

These problems affect all categories in the *DSM*. Most mental disorders have fuzzy boundaries, and fade gradually into normality. When does sadness turn into depression, particularly when life stressors (grief, job loss, breakups of intimate relations) that would upset almost anyone are present? When should anxiety and worry justify diagnosis if there is something real to worry about? At what point is substance use an addiction?

If you do a literature search on overdiagnosis, you won't find much, except articles from Mark Zimmerman's research group. In medicine, emphasis is usually placed on the dangers of underdiagnosis. Of course, no drug company pays you money for warning about overdiagnosis. Also, researchers may be concerned that practitioners are missing their favorite disorder. Epidemiologists are shocked to discover how common mental symptoms are in untreated community populations. Evidently, recognizing that some degree of distress is normal goes against the grain. Yet psychiatry cannot become a clinical science unless it can separate what is pathological from what is normal.

PART II

CATEGORIES MOST LIKELY TO

BE OVERDIAGNOSED

5

HOW MAJOR IS MAJOR

DEPRESSION?

MAJOR DEPRESSION IS ONE OF the most common diagnoses in psychiatry. Constant use over decades has made this category seem as real as myocardial infarction. Yet this category has only been in the *DSM* since 1980, and presents difficult but largely unrecognized diagnostic problems.

Major depression is seriously overdiagnosed. In a recent large-scale survey of clinical practice (Mojtabai, 2013), only 38% of patients who were identified by physicians as having major depression met criteria for the diagnosis. Yet most of them received the same pharmacotherapy as those who did meet *DSM* criteria.

There is a large literature on the problem of under diagnosis of depression (Jacob et al., 2012). However, all these studies describe underdiagnosis of any case that meet *DSM* criteria. This raises the question as to whether clinicians are missing serious depressions that absolutely require treatment, or milder depressions that may not

The more serious problem with major depression is that it is defined in a way that promotes over-recognition. Unfortunately, mental disorders tend to become reified with use (Hyman, 2010). Even so, major depression is not a distinct entity, and is not necessarily "major." The diagnosis describes a heterogeneous group of clinical problems, some of which are severe or even life-threatening, while others derive from the normal vicissitudes of the human condition. Finally, when the requirement is for five out of nine symptoms, many different clinical pictures can be diagnosed in this way.

THE HISTORY OF MAJOR DEPRESSION

The use of the term *major depression* goes back to *DSM-III*. It was an attempt to distinguish episodes with clinically significant effects on functioning from milder symptoms that are temporary and not disabling. Perhaps this is why *DSM-III* and its successors never included a category of *minor* depression. If a patient doesn't meet criteria for the major form, they fall within the realm of adjustment disorders, or possibly depressive disorder, unspecified.

The result is that major depression is a broad category. Anyone with five out of nine symptoms for two weeks can meet criteria for a diagnosis. The short time period and loose criteria make the condition ubiquitous, if not universal. Moffitt et al. (2009) found that at least half of the population will meet criteria for at least one episode over a lifetime.

Patients who might be considered to have minor depression still tend to receive a diagnosis of "major" depression. This practice is based on the assumption that depression is one category, and that clinical presentations vary only according to severity. Traditionally, psychiatrists made a distinction between a severe illness, called melancholia, and episodes of lowered mood that are non-disabling and that are reactions to life circumstances (Parker, 2005). This distinction was removed in *DSM-III*, which supported a unitary theory of depression. An influential article in *Science* by Akiskal and McKinney (1973) argued that there was no basis to separate severe, moderate, and mild depression, and that patients with mild cases could go on to develop more severe forms of the illness. The unitary theory also had a hidden agenda, in that it implied that all patients with major depression should receive the same treatment, that is, antidepressants. It provided an ideological basis for prescribing drugs to people who are unhappy.

The use of the descriptive term *major* has also been used to support the definition of depression as a neurobiological disorder that requires pharmacological treatment. That is the correct view for melancholia. It is not a reasonable view for mild to moderate depression, which is usually an exaggerated response to a loss (Horwitz and Wakefield, 2007). On the one hand, not everyone becomes clinically depressed after a loss (most do not), and genetic vulnerability plays a role in even the most minor depressions (Kendler et al., 1995). Evidence also shows that psychosocial stressors play a causal role in mild to moderate depression (Kendler et al., 1999).

The Harvard psychiatrist Leon Eisenberg (1986) once described a psychiatry that ignores the impact of life events as "mindless." Seeing depression as nothing but a "chemical imbalance" is not even scientific, since the purported imbalances have never been found (Moncrieff and Cohen, 2009). But this widely held belief inevitably leads to intervention on a chemical level, as opposed to the exploration of life histories and active work to develop better coping strategies.

Decades of propaganda from drug companies and their paid consultants from academic psychiatry have reinforced this idea, and have encouraged the view that depression must *always* be treated with antidepressants. There is an important role for psychotherapy in mild to moderate depression, supported by a rich research literature, which also shows that psychological interventions, when successful, can change neurobiology (Beck, 2008). To understand why people become depressed, you have to take life events into consideration, which is exactly what psychotherapy does. Unfortunately, even though the American Psychiatric Association guidelines (2010) suggest that talking therapy can be a first-line intervention, and the NICE guidelines (National Institute for Health and Clinical Excellence, 2011) suggest that talking and support should be tried before prescribing an antidepressant, physicians seem more and more likely to reach for their prescription pad.

The problem with the modern concept of depression is that it downplays psychosocial factors. It is true that even when there are reasons to be depressed, only some people develop symptoms. This outcome depends on both stress and diatheses. But we could attempt to separate cases with a stronger genetic load (which are most likely to need medication) from those with more a more environmental etiology (which may not need medication).

This is the reason that *DSM-III* and *DSM-IV* included a grief exclusion: if depressive symptoms are causally related to a recent loss, one should not make a diagnosis. On the other hand, serious depression that goes on for too long after grief deserves to be considered as a mental disorder. But the exclusion was inconsistent—it does not make sense to focus on grief when so many other adverse life events (e.g., losing intimate relationships, losing a job) can bring on the same symptoms (Wakefield et al., 2007). The decision in *DSM-5* to remove the grief exclusion for diagnosing depression produced controversy, although the manual advises caution about making the diagnosis in such circumstances. The larger question is whether there is really only one form of depression, or a melancholic type and a non-melancholic type. Add to this the temporary periods of unhappiness that meet diagnostic criteria, and depression could have three types—not one.

Debate about the boundaries of major depression misses the proverbial elephant in the room: the overly broad definition of major depression introduced by *DSM-III*. One can receive a diagnosis after suffering as few as five of nine symptoms—for as little as *two weeks*. Although few patients who present clinically will have such a short duration, this drastically brief time scale trivializes the diagnostic construct. It means that almost any bump on life's road can qualify as a depression. A low threshold for diagnosis helps explain why the lifetime prevalence of depression is over 50% (Moffit et al., 2010).

Psychiatry seems to have forgotten that brief periods of sadness in life are normal. Epidemiological research shows such cases usually remit without treatment (Patten, 2008). For this reason, I would have preferred increasing the time scale for a diagnosis to either four or six weeks. Doing so would at least make major depression a little more "major." As it is, we combine under one diagnostic category conditions that need immediate hospitalization, and conditions from which people usually recover on their own.

Prior to 1980, *DSM-II* had distinguished between milder and more severe forms, called neurotic and psychotic depression. Unfortunately, this terminology was problematic. Neurosis had an unclear meaning, which is why it was eventually eliminated from the manual. In addition, severe depression does not always have psychotic features. *DSM-II* attempted to separate depressions that emerge as a severe illness with few triggers from those that are exaggerated reactions to environmental stressors, but it chose the wrong way to make a distinction between mild and severe.

Depression can certainly be divided into the classical melancholia first described by Hippocrates and a less severe syndrome that can affect almost anyone (Parker et al., 2011). Psychiatry had long made use of a separate category of melancholia (Shorter, 2008). The distinction has important clinical implications. When depression comes "out of the blue" and when symptoms are severe, management will almost always include biological intervention (antidepressant drugs with or without adjunctive antipsychotics, electroconvulsive therapy) and/or hospitalization. But when patients are depressed after a loss or a disappointment in life, they can respond to a variety of interventions (psychotherapy, medication, or both), and symptoms often remit spontaneously.

Since the diagnosis of major depression was introduced 35 years ago, many practitioners may not remember that it was once an innovation. Unfortunately, the unitary theory continues to dominate *DSM-5*, which left the construct of major depression unchanged, and only allows clinicians to diagnose melancholia as a subtype or a modifier, not a separate disorder. In contrast, mild depressions can be understood as periods of sadness that mark all lives. These distinctions might be academic if it were not for their impact on treatment choices. The unitary theory of depression, supported by the *DSM* definition, has encouraged unitary therapy. If we required, at the very least, a high score on a scale such as the HAM-D (Hamilton, 1959) as an indication for prescribing, this tendency might be curbed.

SADNESS AND DEPRESSION

Alan Horwitz, a sociologist, and Jerome Wakefield, a social worker, are friends of psychiatry, but they are critical of its diagnostic system. They have published two important books describing the problems of distinguishing between sadness and depression (Horwitz and Wakefield, 2007), and between fear and anxiety (Horwitz and Wakefield, 2012).

In principle, sadness is normal, while depression is pathological. But how can we draw a line between them? Horwitz and Wakefield note that psychiatry has chosen to be over-inclusive rather than under-inclusive. The result is that the diagnostic bar for major depression is too low. When patients come to physicians with sadness, they are likely to receive antidepressant therapy. The proportion of patients receiving these agents who do not have depression is steadily increasing (Mojtabai and Olfson, 2011). This is occurring in spite of evidence that these drugs are not always better than placebo (Kirsch et al., 2008).

Psychiatry is part of modern culture. One of the more striking aspects of our culture is an activist approach to human problems. People do not accept, as they might have in the past, that life can be tragic and marked by disappointment and loss. Yet, as Sigmund Freud once suggested, therapy can only replace neurotic misery with normal human unhappiness.

This attitude toward medical care has been called a wish to be "better than well" (Elliott, 2003). The point of view is very American in spirit, and was openly promoted by Karl Menninger (1963)—an eminent psychiatrist who did, after all, come from Kansas. The wish to be "better than well" is one of the reasons that psychoanalysis was so popular for so long. Like the human potential movement, analysts claimed that everyone could be happy—it just took five years instead of five days to get there.

Psychiatry outside the United States may also not be free of diagnostic inflation—the *International Classification of Diseases* (*ICD*) definition of depression is identical to that in the *DSM*. If physicians could accept the inevitably of sadness, and refuse to pathologize it, the overdiagnosis of depression would be reduced dramatically. But that would require a culture change, not just a change in medical judgment.

ANTIDEPRESSANT EFFECTS AND PLACEBO EFFECTS

Most of my trainees and colleagues believe that any patient with major depression *should* be prescribed an antidepressant, and that these agents are highly effective in both major and minor cases. If the treatment does not work, they change medications, often several times, and/or add another type of drug (usually an antipsychotic).

The evidence does not support these ideas. Antidepressants work best in severely ill patients (although they are sometimes effective in a broader range of cases). This was clearly shown in the widely publicized meta-analysis by Kirsch et al. (2008), which took into account all trials registered with the government, not just the ones that eventually were published in journals. The results were that placebo effects were low in severe depression, but high in mild to moderate depression. Similar findings emerged from a meta-analysis by Fournier et al. (2010). Thus pharmacotherapy has a clear edge in melancholia, but is little better than placebo in many cases seen in outpatient settings.

One might hope that these findings would change practice, and would drive a stake through the heart of the routine prescription of antidepressants. Far from it! The percentage of the US population taking antidepressants has continued to increase, and is now 11% (Pratt et al., 2011). Meanwhile, experts have come up with various reasons that these drugs work better than clinical trials have ever been able to prove (Blier, 2008). Practitioners are understandably reluctant to give up procedures that are a mainstay of their clinical work. And patients, some of whom have been on drugs for years, are afraid to stop taking them. Finally, insurance reimbursement provides a reinforcement for physicians to prescribe these drugs and to keep patients on them.

The perception that if you don't prescribe antidepressants you can be sued for malpractice brings us back to the 1980s and a famous legal case. Raphael Osheroff, a physician, was admitted to a private, psychoanalytically oriented, hospital (Chestnut Lodge in Maryland) and was treated there for six months with psychotherapy alone. His physicians focused on a diagnosis of narcissistic personality disorder (which might also have been present). But they missed the diagnosis of melancholic depression, even though Osheroff spent much of his hospital stay pacing the halls in an agitated state. After being successfully treated with tricyclics at another hospital, the patient sued Chestnut Lodge, and the case was eventually settled out of court. Osheroff went back to his medical practice and lived until 2012. Although no legal precedent was set by this case, the publicity, leading to articles in the *American Journal of Psychiatry* (Klerman, 1990), contributed to a consensus that one should not fail to prescribe antidepressants. Moreover, the generalizability of the Osheroff case is doubtful, since a careful reading of the case material shows that the patient suffered from melancholic depression. The lawsuit was justified, but it cannot be interpreted to mean that failure to prescribe antidepressants automatically puts physicians at legal risk.

Yet standard treatment guidelines adopted by the American Psychiatric Association, most recently revised in 2010, continue to support immediate treatment with antidepressants, whether depression is mild, moderate, or severe, although psychotherapy is acknowledged as an alternative. The British, who often have more common sense than their American colleagues, have a different take on the evidence. The National Institute for Clinical Excellence (NICE, 2009), an independent UK panel not linked to organized psychiatry, publishes guidelines for all of medicine, applying a demanding grid of criteria. NICE specifically recommends that patients with milder forms of depression should *not* be prescribed drugs, but should be followed supportively, and encouraged to improve their lifestyle (e.g., with exercise). Antidepressants are only recommended when these initial interventions fail. And psychotherapy is stated to be an equally effective alternative to drugs.

The NICE guidelines are much more consistent with evidence than the APA recommendations. In line with a "can do" culture, American psychiatrists are more aggressive about treatment. Also, antidepressants are a multibillion-dollar business in the United States, and many prominent psychiatrists have either been co-opted or have had their services bought by the pharmaceutical industry. Many of the experts who sat on APA panels have made millions of dollars by promoting antidepressants. It is hard to believe that profit had no effect on their clinical judgment.

Psychiatrists who follow the recommendations of clinical practice guidelines rarely check to see how strong the evidence is. When I did so for a book (Paris, 2010a), I found that some of the popular alternatives for the treatment of depression, which have been subject to aggressive marketing, had weak research support. For example, augmentation with antipsychotics was supported by only two clinical trials, both paid for by industry, and never independently replicated. Unfortunately, on the grounds that the public should not be denied the benefit of the latest developments in therapeutics, the US Food and Drug Administration (FDA) is satisfied with minimal evidence. And whenever a new FDA "indication" is approved, industry makes sure that the use of drugs will increase dramatically.

In particular, the indication for antipsychotic augmentation suffers from the more general problem of failing to consider the difference between severe and mild to moderate depression. It has long been known that patients with psychotic and melancholic depression need these agents, a practice that goes back to the days of chlorpromazine. It is another matter to prescribe these drugs routinely, particularly to patients with forms of depression that do not even respond well to antidepressants. The only justification might be a need for sedation. However, in a recent press release for the "Choosing Wisely" initiative in medicine (www.choosingwisely.org/apa-releases-list-of-common-uses-of-psychiatric-medications-to-question/), the American Psychiatric Association came out against this practice, on the grounds that less toxic alternatives are better.

Unfortunately, the word has *not* gotten out to clinicians that the medical treatment of major depression suffers from limitations in effectiveness for any drug currently being prescribed. Thus the inappropriate treatment of depression and the failure to consider psychotherapy as an alternative to psychopharmacology follow directly from the overdiagnosis of major depression and the unitary theory.

In summary, the broad concept of major depression reifies the construct of major depression and makes it a bad guideline for management. It also has had the consequence of supporting poorly thought-out screening programs in the community (Patten, 2008). The assumption is that a large number of people are suffering from a treatable illness that could be managed if only they would recognize the problem, consult a physician, and receive antidepressants. This has led to the wide use of screening instruments for use in community populations. People can easily fill out a screener, conclude that they are clinically depressed, and present themselves to a physician for a prescription. Yet most undiagnosed depression in the community is mild, transient, and remitting, and the instruments used to screen for depression are of dubious validity (Thombs et al., 2008). Meanwhile, few psychiatrists need to look for extra work. They could concentrate their efforts on the severely ill patients who would almost certainly benefit from taking antidepressants.

Many patients without depression are being prescribed antidepressants, and while some of these prescriptions may be for anxiety disorders, that would not account for the fact that nearly two-thirds of the sample studied by Mojtabai (2013) had only mild symptoms that did not meet *DSM* criteria. Evidently a large number of people who don't need antidepressants are receiving them anyway. Patients with good reasons to be sad, such as after grief or other losses, are being treated in this way. They may need an entirely different type of intervention. But the diagnostic system is being used to support routine pharmacological intervention.

Failure to consider that antidepressants are not consistently effective for depressive symptoms in practice has led to a wide range of clinical errors. For example, there is a widely held view that antidepressants have a delayed action, and have to be given for at least two weeks, or for two months, before one can say they haven't worked. Yet Posternak and Zimmerman (2005) conducted a meta-analysis showing that patients on placebo have the same delayed response. Moreover, a fair percentage of "treatment-resistant" patients do not respond to antidepressants at all, even after augmentation and switching (Valenstein, 2006).

Clinicians and researchers have also puzzled over the observation that patients receiving a stable dose of antidepressants often stop responding after a few months. Zimmerman and Thongy (2007) showed that this phenomenon can be explained if the populations under study are a mixture of true responders and placebo responders. Thus people who no longer receive benefit from an antidepressant may have only had a placebo response to begin with. And as we have seen, the level of placebo response to these drugs is very high (at least 40%).

Why then do so many *patients* swear by antidepressants? It has been known for many years that people who are demoralized get better if they are provided hope in almost any form (Frank and Frank, 1991). When depressed people go to see a physician, already primed by the media to expect a prescription, and have the belief that medicine will relieve their symptoms, this mechanism is unleashed.

Moreover, once a patient has been taking antidepressants for some time, he or she may well be reluctant to stop them for fear of a relapse. Patients often tell me they had a bad time after forgetting to take their pills for a single day, which actually makes little sense for drugs with an extended half-life.

There is evidence that *some* people need maintenance antidepressants (Hirschfeld, 2000). But that does not mean that everyone who meets criteria for major depression has a lifelong illness requiring lifelong therapy. One reason for the increase in the prevalence of antidepressant use in the population may well be that these drugs are being prescribed on an indefinite basis. They have few serious side effects, and usually do no harm, although women may come for consultation about continuation treatment when thinking about getting pregnant.

The history of medicine is full of treatments that remained popular for decades because almost every practicing physician believed in them. We may look back on some of these stories with dismay, but may not realize that future generations could see some of our present procedures in the same light. I am not suggesting that antidepressants are not effective, but I am saying that their efficacy has been exaggerated, and that these agents should be reserved for severe depression. Because they are easy to prescribe, and because they evoke strong placebo responses, the way they are used today is also a consequence of the overdiagnosis of major depression.

6

BIPOLAR DISORDERS

BIPOLAR DISORDER IS A MAJOR and disabling mental disorder (Goodwin and Jamison, 2007). For this reason, one would expect physicians to diagnose it with some degree of caution. However, its plural form ("bipolar disorders") has come to include a range of variants and related conditions that opens the door to overdiagnosis.

Current diagnostic practice remains based on the dichotomy developed by Emil Kraepelin (1921), distinguishing schizophrenia, a chronic disease affecting cognition with a poorer prognosis, from manic-depression, the older name for an episodic mood disorder with a better prognosis. We are still arguing about the Kraepelinian dichotomy, which has been challenged by recent research (Craddock and Owen, 2005). When psychiatrists are not sure which side of the divide to place a patient, they can use the category *schizo-affective*, but careful study suggests that many of these patients have a more severe form of bipolar disorder (Lake and Hurwitz, 2006), in which psychotic features are more prominent.

Bipolar-II disorder was a new category in *DSM-IV*. Although characterized by hypomania instead of full mania, it usually responds to lithium in the same way as bipolar-I (Parker, 2012). But clinicians need to respect the requirement that hypomania last for at least four consecutive days (usually longer), and that abnormal mood must be continuous. I receive many consultations in which bipolar-II is suspected entirely on the basis of an unstable mood, even when mood swings last for only an hour or two.

The search of occult bipolarity has also affected the evaluation of patients with "treatment-resistant" depressions, who may be thought to be unresponsive because of an underlying bipolar disorder (Sharma et al., 2005). But what is meant by treatment resistance? Patients with mild to moderate depression do not consistently respond to antidepressants. This term should only be applied to severe illnesses, such as melancholia. Second, on what grounds can one determine whether a patient has an underlying bipolar disorder, if its symptoms are absent? We have no biomarkers to help us.

THE BIPOLAR SPECTRUM

The expansion of bipolarity has made overdiagnosis a real danger, and this is already one of the most problematic fads in contemporary psychiatry. In a survey using broad criteria for the bipolar spectrum (Akiskal et al., 2006), based almost entirely on instability of mood, these diagnoses were found in 40% of *all* patients in a psychiatric clinic. The idea that almost half of all patients in psychiatry have occult forms of one disorder can only be seen as an example of what I have called "bipolar imperialism" (Paris, 2012).

What exactly is a bipolar spectrum disorder? The concept assumes that a wide range of patients who receive other diagnoses are "really" suffering from a milder (or variant) form of bipolarity. These views downplay the nonspecificity of mood swings. The main proponents have been the Swiss psychiatrist Jules Angst (1998) and the American psychiatrist Hagop Akiskal (2002). While *DSM-5* has not expanded the definition of bipolar disorders, the tendency to see bipolarity behind every mood swing has had a wide influence on practice. The list of disorders that "imperialists" consider to lie within the bipolar spectrum includes treatment-resistant major depression, substance abuse, and personality disorders (Akiskal, 2002). This makes the spectrum very broad indeed.

It is true that recurrent episodes of severe depression can sometimes convert to bipolarity, but not predictably. In the Akiskal et al. (2006) study, these cases were counted as bipolar spectrum because of the presence of mood swings. And when depression was associated with irritability and impulsivity, Akiskal et al. identified patients as having a bipolar spectrum disorder, even in the absence of hypomanic episodes. Patients with a range of other diagnoses, including substance abuse, eating disorders, and personality disorders, were seen in the same way.

Manic episodes have always been diagnosed on the basis of a triad of symptoms: overactivity, pressure of speech, and elevated mood (Goodwin and Jamison, 2007). Hypomanic episodes are less severe, but *DSM-5* requires that mood be continuously abnormal for at least four days. Mood shifts that do not meet these criteria may or may not be atypical forms of the same illness.

Proving this assumption would require biomarkers as well as an understanding of the endophenotypes behind bipolarity. In their absence, evidence for the concept has mainly depended on family history data (Akiskal, 2002). But it is rare for research reports of family history to be confirmed by informants, and one cannot assume that valid diagnoses can be made on unseen relatives. Yet in the present climate of opinion, patients may be all too ready to report that their relatives were "bipolar." I am only convinced if there has been a history of hospitalization for manic episodes, or (even more strongly) of multiple hospitalizations.

To carry out differential diagnosis of mood symptoms, it is crucial to determine if there has been a clear-cut hypomanic episode. For this purpose, it is very helpful to interview relatives and significant others (Dunner and Tay, 1993). Moreover, to identify an episode, one needs to know its duration, whether mood was consistent or inconsistent, and whether any of the characteristic symptoms of hypomania were present: rapid speech, little need to sleep, excessive spending, and grandiose plans. These are features that other people will notice. Therefore one of the key questions in an interview is to find out whether significant others or coworkers asked patients if something was wrong with them, and observed that they were obviously not their usual self.

Unfortunately, clinicians who have not read the manual closely do not take the time to examine these details. Moreover, it has become common to have a "knee-jerk" reaction to mood instability, either diagnosing bipolar-II, or writing in the notes "rule out bipolar-II." But *DSM-5* does not allow a bipolar diagnosis if patients have never had a hypomanic episode—with one/ important exception. This is the rarely used category of "bipolar disorder, not otherwise specified," now called "bipolar disorder, other specified and unspecified" categories in *DSM-5*. But these diagnoses are not popular in practice, so bipolar-II, incorrectly, occupies the niche.

What might be the real reason for the expansion of the bipolar spectrum? I suggest that it is based on a wish to treat difficult patients with medication. Once one makes diagnoses of bipolar spectrum disorders, mood stabilizers and/or antipsychotics will be prescribed. This accelerates existing trends in the treatment of mood disorders, in that the indications for antipsychotic drugs have been expanded, with many more prescriptions being written (Mojtabai and Olfson, 2010). And, of course, this whole process is driven by overdiagnosis.

BIPOLARITY IN THE PERCEPTIONS OF PATIENTS AND THE PUBLIC

One might think that increases in the pharmacological treatment for mood swings would elicit skepticism from patients, who are, after all, the consumers. Instead, many patients have "bought in" to the bipolar fad. Chan and Sireling (2010) described patients who actually *want* to be bipolar. I have seen quite a few people who are proud of the diagnosis, possibly because their life problems have been explained as due to aberrant chemistry, and thus are not their fault.

The media have also supported an expanded diagnosis of bipolarity. Several celebrities, including movie stars, have publicly stated that they have bipolar-II. On the one hand, we could applaud the reduction of stigma when famous people present themselves as sufferers from mental illness. On the other hand, we don't know if any of these celebrities actually met *DSM-5* criteria for hypomania, or whether they were treated for mood swings with other causes.

The courts have sometimes been impressed by the bipolar spectrum. A prominent Canadian politician who was arrested after stealing an expensive ring had charges dismissed when his psychotherapist informed the court that he had bipolar disorder. This decision was made in spite of the fact that this man was not even on medication. The only consequence he suffered was that he was never re-elected to Parliament.

The diagnosis of bipolarity has even entered our common language. In common parlance, calling someone "bipolar" communicates a perception that a person is moody and difficult. The concept has become rather pervasive, and is now almost as ubiquitous as Freudian terminology was a generation ago—and just as unscientific in its assumptions.

THE HISTORY OF BIPOLARITY

To further understand why bipolar disorder is being diagnosed in people who have never had clear-cut mood episodes, we have to go back in time and examine the history of the disorder. Effective treatment of bipolar disorder was one of the great triumphs of modern psychiatry. Decades ago, Cade (1949) observed cases in which lithium was an effective treatment. Unfortunately, his discovery went unrecognized, in part because lithium was seen as overly toxic. In the 1960s, Mogens Schou, a Danish psychiatrist, conducted systematic trials showing definitively that lithium was effective—and safe if used with caution (Schou, 2001). What followed was one of the greatest of all medical miracles: taking a simple salt to control one of the most disabling of all mental disorders. It was later shown that lithium is the only drug that seems to prevent these patients from dying by suicide (Young and Hammond, 2007).

When I was a medical student, psychiatrists did not have access to lithium. A colleague in Toronto recently told me that in the mid-1960s, after reading scientific papers by Schou, he had a pharmacist prepare lithium carbonate off-label and used it on his most difficult patients. But most psychiatrists treated bipolar patients only with antipsychotics. The problem was that relapse remained common, and these agents could not prevent that from happening, as they usually do in schizophrenia.

In 1970, as a resident, I was the first person to administer lithium at my hospital, to a patient with 25 previous admissions. Once maintenance treatment was established, she never relapsed again. In later years, anti-epileptic drugs became useful alternatives, but they are not as effective as lithium (Geddes et al., 2008). Also, while psychiatrists can usually control bipolar disorder with lithium, it remains a chronic disease. Yet we should not feel too badly—much of modern medicine consists of management, not cure.

A perception has lived on that diagnosing bipolar disorder in more patients will lead to the same miracle cures as in the past. In this way, bipolarity is a victim of its own success. Initially, as psychiatrists rediagnosed psychotic patients who had been considered schizophrenic, they observed sustained recoveries that had not been possible before the introduction of lithium. Research findings also showed that some of the symptoms, particularly those described by the German psychiatrist Kurt Schneider, that had long been considered to be characteristic of schizophrenia were equally common in mania (Abrams and Taylor, 1981).

With time, clinicians were tempted "to offer the benefit of lithium" to more patients. This led them to diagnose a large number of schizophrenic patients as bipolar or schizo-affective. Some got better, but it was hard to tell why, given that admission to hospital uses such a wide range of interventions, and that they were often discharged on five or six drugs. It was not clear whether rediagnosis and new forms of treatment were actually making a difference.

THE ROLE OF INDUSTRY

The pharmaceutical industry can be a partner for medicine, and there is little doubt that many of their discoveries have had positive effects for patients. For example, Eli Lilly deserves credit for pioneering the development of fluoxetine, the first selective serotonin reuptake inhibitor.

The problem is that "Big Pharma" has a different agenda from that of medicine: to make profits for their stockholders. Their vision of an ideal drug is one that would be taken by the largest number of people for the longest time. Industry has therefore been interested in psychiatric conditions that are common in the community, such as mood disorders. Unfortunately, none of the antidepressants developed in the last 25 years is any better than fluoxetine; meta-analyses have found only marginal differences among any of the current options (Cipriani et al., 2009).

Moreover, current marketing encourages physicians and their patients to believe that depression that fails to remit with antidepressant treatment indicates an underlying bipolar disorder, which needs to be treated with other drugs. Promoting this idea to healthcare providers has been bad enough, but direct marketing to patients is much worse. Unfortunately, doing so is legal in the United States (only one other country, New Zealand, allows this). How did it happen?

The pharmaceutical industry was rich enough to effectively lobby members of Congress. The legal change led to advertisements on television, and in magazines, from companies that make mood stabilizers and antipsychotics. They tell people to "ask your doctor" whether you would benefit from a new medication, and whether your symptoms mean that you are not just depressed, but bipolar. This kind of marketing has been a great success, at least for manufacturers.

Meanwhile, the evidence that many patients fail to respond to current agents (Kirsch et al., 2008) hasn't made much of an impression. With pressure from suffering patients, with pharmaceutical representatives coming to the door, and with paid experts from academia promoting the same message, it is not surprising that physicians believe in the practice of aggressive psychopharmacology. The result is that patients who fail to respond to antidepressants are less likely to be referred for psychotherapy, and are more likely to be prescribed antipsychotics and/or anticonvulsant mood stabilizers.

AFFECTIVE INSTABILITY AND BIPOLARITY

Affective instability (AI), also called emotion dysregulation (Linehan, 1993), is one of the main characteristics of patients with borderline personality disorder (BPD). I specialize in the treatment of these patients, who come to me for consultation and/or specialized care. Almost all of them have been told, at some stage, that they have bipolar disorder. This misdiagnosis, which does not actually follow the algorithims in the *DSM* system, has become very common (Ruggero et al.,

2010; Zimmerman et al., 2010). Sometimes a diagnosis of bipolarity is given in the emergency room when patients are agitated and out of control. In that setting, there is usually no time to gather sufficient information to make a firm diagnosis. A diagnosis of bipolarity may also be given in clinics and offices, based on patients' complaints that their moods are "on a roller coaster."

Patients with borderline personality disorder (BPD) have rapid shifts of mood in response to life circumstances, usually in response to interpersonal triggers, and unstable mood has long been considered the crucial feature of the disorder (Linehan, 1993; Siever and Davis, 1991). What you see in BPD are moods that shift by the hour, and that move from depression not to euphoria, but to anger and irritability.

Affective instability (AI) seems to be a separate phenomenon derived from a distinct endophenotype, a conclusion supported by differences both in phenomenology and imaging between patients with bipolar disorder or BPD (Koenigsberg, 2010). Research using ecological momentary assessment (a way of monitoring social interactions in vivo) has shown that rapid mood swings in BPD are a response to negative social interactions, and usually involve anger, not elation (Russell, 1979).

Yet for bipolar imperialists, AI lies on a continuum with classical bipolarity (Akiskal, 2002). One of the strongest arguments against that conclusion is that only a minority of patients with BPD develop true hypomanic episodes, and that unstable mood is actually the most stable clinical feature of these cases (Gunderson et al., 2006). If there are indeed hypomanic episodes, I believe that a diagnosis of bipolar-II should take precedence. Yet when patients with BPD who have AI are viewed as bipolar, they receive the wrong treatment: prescriptions based on a bipolar diagnosis, while evidence for the effectiveness of antipsychotics and mood stabilizers in BPD is weak (Stoffers et al., 2012). Unlike their powerful and convincing effects in classic bipolar illness, these drugs provide only a degree of sedation and never yield a remission of personality disorder symptoms.

Ironically, though clinicians may prefer to diagnose bipolar disorder because they see it as more treatable, it has a worse prognosis than BPD. Borderline personality usually improves as patients get older (Zanarini et al., 2012), while bipolarity does not (Goodwin and Jamison, 2007). Crucially, a diagnosis of a personality disorder allows patients to be referred to evidence-based psychotherapy (Stoffers et al., 2012b).

The problems with overdiagnosis of bipolarity underline the way that medication defines the practice of medicine, so that physicians see their role as writing prescriptions. Psychiatrists may believe that it is hopelessly old-fashioned to carry out psychotherapy, and that real doctors know how to prescribe drugs. Medications are seen as scientific and based on neuroscience, as opposed to "just talking," which evidently is not.

Mojtabai and Olfson (2010) have documented this decline of formal psychotherapy in psychiatric practice. Moreover, patients may not be referred to non-medical health professionals, who now provide almost all psychotherapy services. And the moment a patient is diagnosed with bipolarity, management will be psychopharmacological. If a good number of these patients should actually be diagnosed with a personality disorder, then overdiagnosis is leading to very bad treatment.

PEDIATRIC BIPOLAR DISORDER

The most controversial aspect of the bipolar spectrum has been its expansion into child psychiatry. Since the time of Kraepelin (1921), it was generally accepted that bipolar disorder rarely starts before puberty. Most of the major disorders in psychiatry (schizophrenia, substance abuse, eating disorders, personality disorders) begin in adolescence. All of these conditions have childhood precursors, but symptoms rarely reach clinically significant levels prior to puberty.

Bipolarity tends to be invoked in every area of psychiatry where treatment is difficult. It offers the hope that the drugs that work for classical cases will be effective in other populations. Childhood behavior disorders, especially severe conduct disorder, fit this profile. No one really knows what to do with these children. Psychotherapy rarely makes a dent, and even the best documented approach, Parent Effectiveness Training (Gordon, 2000), has not been shown to be broadly effective. Not surprisingly, frustrated child psychiatrists have turned to drugs for a solution.

The preferred treatment tends to be antipsychotics. These drugs are powerful sedatives, and we often use them in the emergency room, where rapid control of impulsivity is more important than precise diagnosis. But long-term treatment with antipsychotics for behavioral problems in children is an off-label and purely symptomatic indication. If children who are not bipolar are treated for years as if they are, with drugs they do not need, they will endure serious side effects for no good reason.

The evidence base for making bipolar diagnoses in children is thin. There are, however, impulsive children who are also affectively unstable. A long-term study of a cohort of these cases was conducted by Birmhaher et al. (2009). The main finding was that these patients remained affectively unstable into adolescence, but did not develop classical bipolar disorder.

Because the treatment of children is an emotional issue, this is one diagnostic epidemic that has aroused real opposition. *DSM-5*, under the influence of a prominent child psychiatrist, David Shaffer, introduced a new category of disruptive mood dysregulation disorder, specifically designed to reduce the frequency of bipolar diagnoses before puberty (American Psychiatric Association, 2013). Yet this new category is controversial in its own right: it is one of the few new diagnoses in *DSM-5*, and is just beginning to be researched.

MAKING THE MOST OF BIPOLARITY

Instead of expanding the concept of bipolarity, psychiatrists would be better advised to concentrate their efforts on patients who have the classical form of the illness—cases that Emil Kraepelin would have recognized. We are not doing as well with these patients as we had hoped. Bipolar-I disorder has a more serious course than Kraepelin described, sometimes getting worse, not better, with age (Goodwin and Jamison, 2007). Bipolar-II disorder can be a frustrating condition to manage, particularly when the clinical picture is dominated by depression (Parker, 2012). If half the effort that has gone into studying the bipolar spectrum were devoted to developing new and better drugs to manage these patients, everyone would benefit.

7

POST-TRAUMATIC STRESS

DISORDER

DOES TRAUMA CAUSE PTSD?

Trauma and stress are universal human experiences. Since Homer's *Odyssey*, it has been recognized that people can suffer long-term psychological effects from having been in extreme danger. The diagnosis of post-traumatic stress disorder (PTSD) medicalizes and validates this kind of distress. However, this construct is of recent vintage, having only been introduced in 1980.

Interest in PTSD has mainly been sparked by war and terrorism, but has also been fueled by interest in phenomena such as rape and armed robbery. When we encounter survivors of these adversities, we tend to have an emotional response, sympathizing with victims, and thinking "that could have been me."

Our reaction to other people's traumas has made some people assume that trauma usually causes PTSD, or that a wide range of psychiatric symptoms are trauma-related. Actually, there is no predictable relationship between adversity and the development of symptoms. Most people exposed to trauma will never develop PTSD. Trauma is a trigger, but not a sufficient cause, of PTSD (McNally, 2003).

Instead, vulnerability determines who develops and who does not develop the disorder. Trait neuroticism, that is, the tendency to become easily upset and to remain upset, is a more important predictor than trauma itself (Breslau et al., 1991). This follows a more general principle: mental disorders do not result from single causes, but from interactions between multiple risk factors (Uher and Rutter, 2012).

Failure to recognize the complexity of the pathways to psychopathology is one factor in the overdiagnosis of PTSD. The human mind is programmed to look for cause and effect, and even the youngest children make causal attributions (Bloom, 2004). But all too often, linear explanations of complex phenomena lead to sloppy thinking.

THE DIAGNOSIS OF PTSD

Younger clinicians may be surprised to learn that PTSD was included in the *DSM* only after a lengthy political struggle, and that its history has been complex (Young, 1997). Clinical descriptions of symptoms following trauma go back to the US Civil War. "Shell shock" was a topic of interest during World War I, and was called "combat exhaustion" in World War II. *DSM-I*, published seven years after that war, included a category of "gross stress reaction," which extended these concepts to civilian trauma. But that construct was narrower than PTSD, and did not attract research interest. The diagnosis was dropped in *DSM-II*, which was published during the Vietnam War. Ironically, in 1968, it was thought that rapid intervention could prevent the development of symptoms. However, when a large number of Vietnam veterans presented to hospitals with symptoms related to war experiences, psychiatrists who worked with this clientele put pressure on the American Psychiatric Association to include a diagnosis related to traumatic exposure. In response, the current concept of PTSD was developed, and it was included in *DSM-III*.

While exposure to deadly combat drove PTSD, war veterans often had problems like substance abuse and depression that were not necessarily related to their service and had been present prior to their time in the military (Young, 1997). It was also established that some patients receiving treatment for service-related PTSD in the US Veterans Administration (VA) system had never been in combat (McNally, 2007). However, this diagnosis provided a convenient way to provide treatment for patients in these hospitals.

It requires clinical judgment to determine whether presenting symptoms are causally related to a traumatic event. Israeli researchers (Zohar et al., 2009) found that most soldiers do not develop PTSD, even after the most severe combat exposure. PTSD was more common in American soldiers going to Iraq than it was in British soldiers (Hotopf et al., 2006). It is true that the British saw less combat, and that intensity of combat is a strong predictor of later symptoms (Iversen et al., 2007). But it is also possible that American psychiatrists and psychologists are more likely to make the diagnosis, and that British soldiers still have a stiff upper lip

In civilian trauma, prospective studies of Australian firefighters (McFarlane, 1989) and of large community populations (Breslau et al., 1991) have found that most PTSD patients had prior vulnerabilities, such as a high level of neuroticism or past traumas. Thus adverse events are a "tipping point" for people whose adaptation is already fragile.

The definition of PTSD was more specific than its predecessors in that it described three characteristic features that *had* to be present: persistent re-experiencing of the event, avoidance of stimuli associated with a trauma, and symptoms of increased arousal. Unfortunately, clinicians have not always been systematic in applying these criteria. They may *want* to diagnose PTSD, perhaps because doing so opens the door to accessible treatment. In the Veterans Administration system, psychotherapy is free. Where I work, in the Canadian single payer system, although coverage for psychiatry is free, psychotherapy by non-psychiatrists is not well insured. But if you are beaten up, raped, or hit by a car, the government will pay for a year of therapy with a psychologist—if it can be established that PTSD is the diagnosis.

Social forces also play a role in the wish to diagnose PTSD. During the unpopular Vietnam War, therapists who opposed the war were eager to show that it was seriously harming soldiers who participated. Young (1997), an anthropologist, wrote a widely cited book describing his observations in a large hospital. He concluded that services were so extensive that the system encouraged some veterans to remain disabled.

Many of the same principles apply to civilian trauma. A "culture of victimhood" has had a good deal of influence on contemporary society (Furedi, 2003). Some of these phenomena are relatively trivial, such as people talking about their personal traumas on television, or biographies of famous people becoming "pathographies" in which unhappy childhoods are invoked to explain troubled lives. Others are more malignant, such as a clinical vogue for uncovering "repressed memories" (McNally, 2003), and the imprisoning of day-care workers for fictional crimes against children (McHugh, 2005). The power of cultural forces becomes apparent to anyone who questions a diagnosis of PTSD, which involves a risk of being accused of failing to validate human suffering.

OVERDIAGNOSING PTSD

Overdiagnosis of PTSD is the result of careless thinking and emotional bias. Failing to determine whether the patient actually meets criteria for the disorder, as listed in the manual, seems to be common. (Mark Zimmerman's MIDAS project has not yet examined this question.) If there is a traumatic event in a patient's history, it may automatically be assumed to be the cause of current symptoms. Other diagnoses may be more relevant, and it may not add much to put PTSD on the list. Yet diagnosing PTSD can be seen as a necessary validation of a patient's suffering.

PTSD is almost the only disorder in the *DSM* that evokes, rightly or wrongly, a specific etiology. But trauma is only a risk factor for PTSD, not a definitive cause. The disorder only develops when adverse life experiences touch on temperament and vulnerability. This principle, the stress-diathesis model (Monroe and Simons, 1991), states that neither stress nor diathesis alone is a sufficient condition for developing mental disorders.

This model can be applied to a long-standing controversy about the "A criterion" for PTSD in the *DSM* system, which defines the nature of the traumatic event to which a patient has been exposed (McNally, 2009). This criterion is broad enough to describe almost any stressor or adverse life event, and was expanded in both *DSM-IV* and *DSM-5*.

The A criterion has now come to include not only those who have been directly exposed, but also those who have been witnesses, as well as those who have only learned about an event (Rosen et al., 2008; McHugh and Treisman, 2007). This was a bad decision. There is no good evidence that this expanded list of experiences constitute important risk factors for PTSD (McNally and Breslau, 2008). For example, after 9/11, some worried that a large percentage of the population might develop PTSD from watching traumatic events on television. However, as shown by a longitudinal study (Breslau, Bohnert, Bohnert, and Koenen, 2010), the actual rate in people with indirect exposure to the 9/11 events was 0.3%, and even that may have had nothing to do with the "trauma."

PTSD should be restricted to symptoms resulting from direct exposure to life-threatening trauma. And using the current definition, it must last for at least six months. Many people suffer short-term symptoms after traumatic exposure that remit with time. In that case, the diagnosis is not PTSD, but "acute stress reaction." In contrast to that quasi-normal reaction, PTSD is a chronic disease that emerges from interaction between exposure, inborn vulnerabilities, and past traumas.

PTSD has become a symbol and a cultural artifact of the modern world. Is the diagnosis more common in some cultures than in others, or is it just more likely to be diagnosed in some cultures than others? Furedi (2003) suggests that PTSD can be an example of "therapy culture," a perspective in which all of life's vicissitudes are medicalized and are seen as treatable.

The diagnosis of PTSD remains problematic because it confounds a putative etiological factor with a typical set of symptoms. North et al. (2009) concluded that PTSD is a syndrome that is cohesive in clinical characteristics, biological correlates, familial patterns, and longitudinal diagnostic stability, but that some symptoms (avoidance and numbing) are more specific to the syndrome, while others are much more nonspecific. Failure to ensure that these symptoms are present is sadly frequent, and one of the most common tendencies is to ascribe causality to life events, even when they are temporally distant.

Unlike some of the other diagnostic epidemics described in this book, the overdiagnosis of PTSD has *not* been driven by a wish to prescribe medication. SSRIs have been used to provide symptomatic relief for anxiety (Brady et al., 2000), and some studies have examined memory-altering drugs such as propanolol (Cukor et al., 2009). But while symptomatic treatment can sometimes be helpful, no drug is specific for PTSD.

The driving force behind the concept and the wish to identify PTSD comes from psychotherapists, many of whom see trauma as a central issue for their practice. When psychiatrists make a diagnosis, they are likely to make a referral to a psychologist. Cognitive behavioral therapy (CBT), particularly the use of exposure techniques, has long been used for PTSD (Rauch et al., 2012). Claims for the superiority of other methods (such as Eye Movement Desensitization Retraining) have not been supported by research (Seidler and Wagner, 2006).

The overdiagnosis of PTSD can put patients at some risk of receiving inappropriate treatment. Under the influence of psychoanalysis, the idea was long current that many patients suffered from childhood traumatic events, which they had either forgotten or had failed to process. While there can be a grain of truth in this idea in some patients, therapists need to focus on the present, and on the sensitivity to life events that produces and maintains symptoms. Therapy works by learning new skills that can be used in one's current life; focusing too much on the past is usually counterproductive.

Even therapies that focus on processing more recent trauma can miss some important points. The problem with such interventions is that they fail to address the vulnerability that makes people over-react to life events. Patients need, above all, strategies to manage responses to adversity, supported by the observation that standard CBT is as good as trauma-specific therapy (Seidler and Wagner, 2006). Any diagnosis of PTSD in patients is likely to be associated with high levels of neurotic personality traits (Breslau et al., 1991), and many patients can also be diagnosed with other anxiety disorders or with depression.

This is why the enthusiasm for diagnosing PTSD over the last several decades has not done much for patients' functioning. Moreover, the population meeting criteria for the diagnosis is heterogeneous. Some have suffered an acute trauma that produces symptoms on its own. Others have long-term problems, with trauma as the tipping point, and are therefore less likely to respond to treatment methods that focus on specific life events. Also, we do not have enough long-term follow-up data on this population to determine the extent to which treatment makes a difference in outcome over time. The key question is whether focusing on adverse events takes proper account of a patient's life history.

Another problem with PTSD is that it often seems that you can't raise questions about the diagnosis without facing political criticism. If you question the meaning of this category in veterans, you can be accused of lacking respect for those who were prepared to give their life for their country. If you raise questions about PTSD in refugees, you may be told you do not understand the conditions under which people live in war-torn and poverty-stricken countries. At a scientific meeting I attended a few years ago, one of the best-known researchers on PTSD was attacked, largely because of her position that it cannot be accounted for by traumatic events alone.

PTSD runs the danger of encouraging victimhood and discouraging a sense of responsibility for one's life. The debate about this diagnosis is not just a matter of evaluating empirical data, but about society's concern over oppression and suffering. That cannot be good for psychiatry, which must put science ahead of politics.

8

ATTENTION DEFICIT

HYPERACTIVITY DISORDER

THE MEDICALIZATION
OF ATTENTION

Many people have trouble maintaining attention, and we all do from time to time. Some of us take stimulants that do not require a prescription. The most universal is caffeine, either in the stronger dose found in coffee, or the weaker one found in tea. Nicotine is also a stimulant, and while its use has declined, it has hardly died out. Taking any of these agents is a personal choice, and need not be based on a medical diagnosis.

The use of amphetamine and amphetamine-like stimulants is another matter. These agents require a prescription, which has to be based on a definite diagnosis. This is how problems in attention became medicalized, and why new diagnoses to justify the use of stimulants had to be developed.

The medicalization of attention also reflects changes in society over the last century. Schoolchildren are not allowed to drop out early and go to work, but are expected to sit at their desks and concentrate for long periods. College students are under pressure to maintain high performance.

Ambitious adults must master tasks that require sustained attention and multitasking. These social demands may have fueled patient requests for stimulants.

Amphetamine was first discovered in 1887, but its use as a drug dates from the 1930s, a time when there were few pharmacological alternatives for the treatment of depression (Shorter, 2008). However, it was quickly recognized that amphetamines have troublesome autonomic side effects, and that they can be habituating, if not addictive. Methylphenidate (Ritalin), considered less dangerous, was introduced in 1955 as a drug to treat hyperactivity in children, and was later used for inattention. But it took another 40 years for this drug, and its pharmacological relatives, to become popular stimulants for adults who experience problems with attention and focusing in their daily life.

A DIAGNOSTIC EPIDEMIC

Attention deficit hyperactivity disorder (ADHD) is one of the most striking diagnostic epidemics of our times. When a disorder increases so rapidly in prevalence, you have to question the validity of the criteria for its diagnosis. Psychopathology doesn't change rapidly over time, and increased recognition of a clinical problem cannot account for doubling, tripling, or quadrupling of prevalence over a few years. Currently the Center for Disease Control (2011) estimates that 11% of all schoolchildren meet criteria for ADHD. Kessler et al. (2006) estimated the prevalence of adult ADHD to be 4.4%. These large numbers are not the result of a scientific breakthrough. They reflect diagnostic inflation, an artificial and faddish inflation of community prevalence.

When I was a student, we diagnosed cases of ADHD, but it was considered an uncommon syndrome. Children with behavioral problems were usually classified as having conduct disorder. It was also assumed that hyperactivity declines with maturity, and the diagnosis of ADHD was unheard of in adults.

The use of amphetamine for behavior problems in children was first described in 1937 (Lange et al., 2010), but it was replaced by methylphenidate in the 1950s. As a resident in child psychiatry in 1970, I prescribed this drug for a condition that *DSM-II* called "hyperkinetic disorder of childhood." A renamed diagnosis of attention deficit disorder (ADD) appeared in *DSM-III* in 1980, and was a broader concept that focused on attention rather than on hyperkinesis alone. In *DSM-III-R*, in a development that later proved crucial, an inattentive subtype was added to the hyperactive type, leading to the renaming of the condition as attention-deficit hyperactivity disorder (ADHD).

One factor promoting the diagnosis, in both childhood and adulthood, is the existence of community groups. The most important is Children and Adults with Attention-Deficit Hyperactivity Disorder (CHADD), a nonprofit organization devoted to advocacy for ADHD diagnosis and treatment. The organization publishes a glossy journal, *Attention*, devoted to their cause. Notably, the funding of CHADD comes from Ciba-Geigy, the company that manufactures Ritalin.

ADHD IN CHILDREN

The ADHD diagnosis is driven by the use of stimulants. There is no doubt that these drugs help children with classical cases of ADHD, particularly the hyperactive subtype, although not all patients respond to them (Leung and Lemay, 2003). It is also possible that inconsistency of response could be due to other conditions that produce a similar clinical picture.

ADHD, like most disorders in psychiatry, is a syndrome, not a disease. The claim by Faraone (2005) that this diagnosis fulfills all Robins-Guze criteria for validity is very doubtful. In children, it cannot be easily separated from conduct disorder, and both course of illness and response to treatment are highly variable (Bishop and Rutter, 2009). Moreover, like other mental disorders, ADHD lacks biomarkers. While a few neuroimaging findings can be associated with this clinical picture (Durston, 2003), they are not specific.

Finally, as pointed out by Shah and Morton (2013), ADHD measures traits that are continuous with normality. In the case of hypertension, research has been carried out to determine at what level traits become clinically significant and meet criteria for a disorder. The current definition of ADHD fails to do the same thing, and the threshold it suggests is arbitrary.

With a less than precise definition, it is not surprising that estimates of the prevalence of ADHD have been very high, even if they are not quite consistent. For example, it has been estimated that 5%–6% of schoolchildren meet current diagnostic criteria (Faraone et al., 2000; Parens and Johnstone, 2009), but the Centers for Disease Control (2011) suggest that the prevalence is 11%, more than twice as much. Both could be overestimating the number of cases that cause clinically significant dysfunction.

Rutter and Uher (2012) comment that ADHD is not always a problem in its own right, and that children tend to be referred when they have a comorbid conduct disorder.

This may be why research in Europe consistently shows lower rates than in the United States (Faraone et al., 2000). Is the difference due to Americans looking for it more, or due to Europeans being more cautious? For Faraone et al. (2003), cross-national differences only mean that if other countries diagnose ADHD less frequently, they are missing it, and that clinicians around the world need to be trained to identify more cases. This circular argument ignores that the fact that there is no gold standard for the diagnosis of ADHD. That kind of reasoning promotes diagnostic epidemics.

As more children are prescribed stimulants, ADHD has become a catch-all diagnosis for disruptive behavior disorders (conduct disorder, and its less severe variant, oppositional defiant disorder). We have seen a similar process in bipolar disorder, in which classic cases are often lithium-sensitive, while spectrum cases are generally not. Classic melancholic depression is another example: it responds to antidepressants in a fairly predictable way, not seen in mild to moderate cases. It is possible that when biomarkers are discovered for ADHD, they will identify a narrower group of patients who do well with stimulants, separating them from other conditions with a phenomenological resemblance.

There has always been a degree of controversy about the ADHD diagnosis. Some of the opposition comes from those with a "knee-jerk" bias against the prescription of drugs to children. But the most informed criticism concerns the boundaries of the diagnosis. Are patients who do not have ADHD being prescribed stimulants?

A large-scale epidemiological survey (Angold et al., 2000) found that 28% of children who meet criteria for ADHD were not on medication, but that 5% of children who did not meet criteria for ADHD (a very large number) nonetheless received stimulants. Since this study was conducted 15 years ago, the picture might look even worse today.

In summary, there are several problems with the ADHD diagnosis, which are also found in many other conditions in psychiatry. They include lack of specificity, unclear boundaries, and the absence of biomarkers. The issue is not whether ADHD in children is a valid diagnosis; like depression, it is a phenomenon that, at an extreme, interferes with functioning. The question is whether children with other kinds of behavioral dysfunction are receiving this diagnosis, and are being treated as if they resembled classical cases. And since stimulants increase focus and attention in everyone, we cannot use treatment response as a validator. Moreover, ADHD, which has no biomarkers (Singh, 2008), may be, at least in part, a result of relatively modern societal expectations for children.

While all these issues should make clinicians cautious, enthusiasm for both diagnosis and treatment has dramatically spread. And when a child is diagnosed with ADHD, it is often suggested to parents that they too could suffer from the same condition. It is true that there is behavioral genetic evidence for a heritable factor in ADHD. But that is insufficient to conclude that it affects first-degree relatives like a Mendelian dominant.

ADULT ADHD

It has been shown by follow-up research that some children outgrow the symptoms of ADHD, but that many do not (Weiss and Hechtman, 2002). A view has therefore developed that ADHD can be a lifelong disease. And when adults have attention problems, they may be retrospectively diagnosed as having had the disorder during childhood.

DSM-5 specifically requires that ADHD cannot be diagnosed in adults without a childhood history of the disorder. *DSM-5* has now extended the age of onset to before 12 (it previously had to be before age 7). Also, while some adults who seem to meet criteria have been diagnosed and treated with stimulants as children, others have not, and many with attention problems complain about them for the first time as adults. Yet given the vast increase in diagnosis among children over the last few decades, one might expect that fewer cases were missed earlier.

It is very easy for adults to become convinced that they currently have ADHD, and therefore must have always had it. Perhaps one's job proves more difficult than expected, particularly if it requires multitasking. Or perhaps a child has received the diagnosis, and the message is given out that this is a genetic disorder than runs strongly in families. In these cases, one is tempted to think back on one's childhood in a new way. Characteristics that were considered normal developmental bumps become redefined in memory as the early features of a neurodevelopmental disorder.

Sometimes this perception is encouraged by well-meaning physicians. Moreover, ADHD has become part of our culture. Anybody who has trouble focusing will consider this possibility. If your friends and relatives say that you might have the condition, and if an Internet search seems to confirm it, you may well consult a doctor to ask if you need stimulants. The answer is likely to be yes. Physicians want to please their patients and to help them, feeling that there is nothing to lose by a medication trial. Once initiated, it is very difficult to determine whether stimulants are working. Like all medications in psychiatry, they have a powerful placebo effect. Add to that the long-established fact that stimulants improve attention in normal people as well (Rapoport et al., 1978).

The category of adult ADHD, as currently defined, was accepted in *DSM-III*, and the adult form of ADHD was first listed as a separate diagnosis in *DSM-IV*. For a few years, adult ADHD was still seen as uncommon. Then, its prevalence in the population as a whole was estimated by a large-scale epidemiological study at 4% (Kessler et al., 2006). This very high number has been used to justify devoting major resources to the problem. At the same time, the adult form has become the subject of a large body of research (Barkley, 2006).

The question is not whether attention problems in adults are real, but whether they can only be explained in this way. Patients with adult ADHD have widespread comorbidity, particularly with personality disorders (Cumyn et al., 2009). Thus adult ADHD may be a real syndrome whose prevalence is over-estimated by including patients whose problems with attention have other causes (depression, anxiety, substance abuse, personality disorder). But attention problems of any kind can receive an ADHD diagnosis, and the *DSM-5* criteria are not specific enough to discourage this practice.

Overdiagnosis (and the use of stimulants that inevitably follows an ADHD diagnosis) has been aggressively promoted by the pharmaceutical industry. The prescription of stimulants to adults has gone up dramatically in recent years (Olfson et al., 2013). These drugs are attractive to physicians, who want to do something for their patients. They are also popular with the general public, some of whom have become greatly attached to their diagnosis. You wouldn't expect dramatic results from prescribing stimulants to a heterogeneous group of patients. Yet evaluation of outcome is muddled by the fact that *everyone's* attention is better on stimulants, so that adult patients, unlike children, may want to take these drugs, and are reluctant to stop them.

Allen Frances has expressed regret about including adult ADHD in *DSM-IV* (Batstra and Frances, 2012). There was evidence at the time supporting that decision, which reflected a consensus, rightly or wrongly, in the clinical and research communities. But no one realized that it opened the door to a diagnostic epidemic.

One cannot diagnosis adult ADHD with a blood test or a scan, and evaluation depends entirely on the clinical assessment of signs and symptoms. While many people seem to believe that psychological testing provides a firm basis for identifying this condition, they are sadly mistaken. In the absence of a gold standard, all that neuropsychological testing can do is to describe problems in more detail—this procedure does not discriminate ADHD from alternative diagnoses.

Moreover, some physicians are not aware that adult ADHD cannot be diagnosed without a history of having the disorder in childhood. To determine in an adult patient whether ADHD was a problem during childhood, one has to ask the patient to remember events of his or her childhood that occurred 15 or more years earlier. It can be helpful to examine school records. Yet outside specialized clinics, few have the time to do that. One can ask patients whether they were in trouble in primary school, or whether they were ever taken out of class. But of course there could be many reasons for that. Even if there is no such history, the claim that problems were not picked up is a retrospective perception, fitting distant memories of childhood into a story.

Part of the story of ADHD overdiagnosis derives from the pharmaceutical industry. There are vast profits to be made by getting large numbers of people to take amphetamine and its pharmacological variants. In December 2013, the *New York Times* published an article by Alan Schwarz showing how clever advertising has been used to promote the prescription and sales of stimulants, both to children and adults, for putative diagnoses of ADHD. The most interesting part of this story was that Keith Connors, the psychologist who created the standard scale for identifying ADHD in children, stated he was concerned as everyone else about the problem. As Connors put it, the rising rates of ADHD diagnosis are "a national disaster of dangerous proportions."

In summary, the overdiagnosis of ADHD, like that of so many other disorders in psychiatry, is a scandal built on good intentions. We need to know more about the syndrome, but current practice is not rooted in science. Those with an interest in the history of psychiatry may be aware that stimulants (often used along with barbiturates) were a mainstay for the management of anxiety and depression some 60 years ago (Shorter, 2008). Just like today, students also took stimulants to do better on their exams, and there was a brisk trade in drugs that were not prescribed for those who used them. Of course, all stimulants were originally prescribed for patients who came to physicians with a variety of psychological symptoms. Now we look back on these practices as at least poorly thought out, or at most primitive. How much better are we doing today?

DIFFERENTIAL DIAGNOSIS OF ADHD

Attention is a basic cognitive function that has attracted much research and that can be affected by a wide variety of mental disorders (Posner, 2012). ADHD is only one of these, and as we have seen, the diagnosis is only a rough approximation of a very complex set of pathways to psychopathology.

First, attention is negatively affected by depression (deRaedt and Koster, 2010). When mood is low, so will be focus and productivity. This is obvious, yet chronically depressed patients are sometimes prescribed stimulants. As discussed in Chapter 5, one answer lies in the concept of "treatment resistance." When patients do not respond to antidepressants, as happens fairly regularly in practice, physicians may ask themselves whether the problem is "really" ADHD. Moreover, patients can be receptive to the option of taking stimulants, and may even see short-term benefits due to the nonspecific effects of these agents.

A second possibility is that anxiety disorders can cause deficits in attention. While state anxiety creates attentional bias (the tendency to over-perceive danger), trait anxiety interferes with the executive functioning that is necessary for attentional focus (Pacheco-Unguetti et al., 2010). Thus chronic anxiety, which can be seen in many disorders, can mimic some features of ADHD.

A third and frequent issue is that patients with personality disorders (PDs) can have attentional deficits. This has been shown in antisocial personality disorder (Black et al., 2010), as well as in borderline personality disorder (Baer et al., 2012). Although not formally documented in other PDs, problems in attention and focus are common in people whose work and relationships suffer from dysfunction over long periods. However, since personality disorder does not have an effective pharmacological treatment, physicians may avoid making such diagnoses.

All these "comorbidities" have long been known (Biederman et al., 1991), but may be seen as subgroups of ADHD, as opposed to alternative diagnoses that account for attention problems through a different pathway. When clinicians are looking for attention deficits, they can find them—they are almost everywhere in clinical practice! This is a good example of a confirmation bias (Kahnemann, 2011). If you believe that ADHD is very common but insufficiently recognized, you will easily travel down the path to overdiagnosis.

9

PERSONALITY AND

PERSONALITY DISORDER

NORMAL PERSONALITY

People are different, and each of us has a unique personality profile. The term *personality* describes these individual differences in thinking, emotion, and behavior. The term *personality disorder* (PD) describes what happens when personality is dysfunctional, leading to serious problems in work and relationships.

A very large empirical literature, based on self-report measures, quantifies the traits that define normal personality differences. This research, largely based on what is called the Five-Factor Model (FFM; Widiger and Costa, 2013) describes domains of (1) neuroticism, (2) extraversion, (3) openness to experience, (4) agreeableness, and (5) conscientiousness. Thus, people can be more or less "neurotic" (i.e., easily upset and sensitive), more extraverted or introverted, open or closed to experience, agreeable or disagreeable, and conscientious or impulsive.

This model has dominated research in trait psychology for the last several decades. It may not be ideal, but it is the most studied. Even so, the model has limitations. First, the FFM was validated in community populations, not in patients, and does not cover the same ground as diagnoses of personality disorder. In spite of the claim that trait dimensions are continuous with personality (Costa and Widiger, 2013), severe disorders have many features not seen in community populations. Second, any method of assessment based on self-report questionnaire will not always correspond to clinical ratings or to peer assessments. Third, no biomarkers are associated with any trait dimensions.

The crucial issue is where normal personality ends and PD begins. PDs are defined in *DSM-5* as abnormalities in cognition, emotion, and behavior that characterize individuals, in many situations, and over extended periods of time. But we all have personality traits that get us into difficulty. (If you don't know what they are, just ask your family or your friends.) So how do we draw the line between normal and abnormal?

Since PD can be understood, at least in part, as an amplified and dysfunctional result of normal trait profiles, many psychologists have favored a dimensional classification of PDs. One suggestion is to score profiles using the Five-Factor Model (Costa and Widiger, 2013). However, the PD research community is divided between those who study severe PDs, preferring categories that describe these disabling disorders, and those who study personality traits, preferring dimensions that blend into normality. *DSM-5* has retained a categorical system, although it had considered (but eventually rejected) a proposal for combining categories and dimensions in a hybrid system (Skodol, 2010, 2011a, 2011b). This system can now be found in Section III of the manual, which is devoted either to alternative models or to conditions requiring further study.

CATEGORIES OF PERSONALITY DISORDER

A diagnosis of personality disorder is based on a serious level of dysfunction in work and relationships that is related to traits, and to the symptoms that dysfunctional traits can produce. There is no sharp cutoff between personality and PD (Livesley et al., 1998), but severe PDs have dramatic symptoms that almost everyone would agree are due to a serious mental disorder. The two categories that stand out are also the most researched.

The first is antisocial personality disorder (ASPD). We know a lot about this condition, even if we have no way of treating it. As shown many years ago (Robins, 1966), ASPD starts in childhood as severe conduct disorder, and the adult diagnosis is a continuation of a pattern of impulsivity, irresponsibility, and callousness. It is important to make this diagnosis, even if doing so doesn't lead to therapy, since we need to avoid unnecessary interventions.

Since there is no effective treatment, ASPD is more likely to be underdiagnosed than overdiagnosed. I have seen cases where patients with ASPD turn up in the emergency room, often under the influence of substances, and are diagnosed and treated as psychotic or "bipolar" on the basis of behavioral dyscontrol and agitation. So it is a good idea to explore life histories and to find out whether patients have ever had contact with the legal system.

The other diagnosis that almost everyone agrees is a mental disorder is borderline personality disorder (BPD). These patients are emotionally labile, have unstable relationships, and often come to treatment after cutting and/or overdosing (Biskin and Paris, 2012). About half hear voices from time to time. The full clinical picture is unmistakable. This has not prevented clinicians who favor a bipolar diagnosis from seeing all BPD patients as falling within that "spectrum" (Ruggero et al., 2010). It also has not prevented clinicians from diagnosing a comorbid depression, entirely missing the PD. In practice, misdiagnosis is very common.

It is important to diagnose BPD because effective treatments have been developed that are specific to the condition (Paris, 2008b). If you think a borderline patient is bipolar, you will prescribe a lot of drugs that don't work, and will fail to offer the psychotherapies that have been shown to be effective.

ASPD and BPD are easy to separate from normal personality because they have striking behavioral features. Of course, people can be callous and manipulative without meeting criteria for ASPD, and not every patient who overdoses has BPD. Nonetheless, when life trajectories are properly assessed, patients with these disorders are very different from the people in your life that give you trouble.

THE PREVALENCE OF PERSONALITY DISORDERS

Because PDs can blend into normality, it is difficult to determine their prevalence. The Epidemiological Catchment Area Study (Robins and Regier, 1991), the first survey to look at

DSM-defined disorders in the community, didn't even try. The only category it measured was ASPD, since it could be identified by a striking behavioral pattern. The National Comorbidity Study (NCS; Kessler et al., 1997), the next generation of research, did much the same. However, the National Comorbidity Study Replication (NCS-R; Kessler et al., 2005b), conducted about a decade later, examined the prevalence of all the *DSM*-defined personality disorders. The overall prevalence was 10%, with nearly 3% for ASPD and a little less than 1% for BPD (Lenzenweger et al., 2007).

Most PDs were assessed for prevalence in an even larger-scale study, the National Epidemiological Survey on Alcohol and Related Conditions (NESARC; Grant et al., 2004b), originally designed to determine the prevalence of substance abuse. However, the numbers it reported were problematic (Paris, 2010c). As in previous studies, NESARC made diagnoses using checklists administered by research assistants (not clinicians). But diagnosing PDs requires experience and judgment. A later re-analysis of the data, using more conservative criteria, brought the overall prevalence down by about half (Trull et al., 2010). Even so, these numbers are still higher than most other researchers have found (Lenzeweger et al., 2007; Coid et al., 2006).

A good example of the problem of separating disorders from traits was that in the NESARC study, the most common PD was obsessive-compulsive, with a prevalence of 7%. Even if the criteria for that diagnosis were valid, all these numbers indicate is that 7% of us are unusually scrupulous and perfectionistic. These are traits that work well in many contexts, and don't necessarily define a mental disorder. As much as I love my own sub-specialty, I am opposed to diagnosing too many people with a PD.

NESARC's numbers would have been even higher if they had included personality disorder, not otherwise specified (PD-NOS, called "other specified" or "unspecified" in *DSM-5*). This can be the most prevalent PD in clinical settings (Zimmerman et al., 2005). The diagnosis simply reflects the fact that patients who meet overall criteria for a PD often don't fit into any of the specific categories listed in the *DSM*.

It is easy to believe that 10%–15% of the population are seriously unhappy, or are good at making other people unhappy. That is human nature—we all have traits that work against us. But inflated prevalence of PDs undermines the concept of disorder, as it does for all mental illnesses. If you define life as psychopathology, is psychiatry the cure?

The main problem for practice is the converse: PD is too often dismissed or ignored. The five-axis system of *DSM-III* and *DSM-IV*, which was designed to focus clinical attention on personality through Axis II, didn't help. How many times have you seen a clinical note with an Axis I diagnosis, followed by "Axis II, deferred?" If you don't want to take personality into account, and prefer to diagnose mood and anxiety disorders, that is what you will write down. With this problem in mind, the decision of *DSM-5* to drop Axis II was the right one.

The preference for symptomatic disorders, as opposed to long-term interpersonal dysfunction, also reflects a wish to prescribe medication. Patients with PDs who have depressive symptoms, particularly in the case of BPD, are often seen as suffering from a mood disorder. And if mood is unstable, then bipolarity may be considered. Yet research fails to support the idea that BPD is a mood disorder, which, as originally defined by Kraepelin (1921), describes an episode in which patients are not functioning as their normal self.

When a mood episode is over, patients "become themselves" once again. In contrast, a personality disorder describes a self that is itself abnormal, affecting psychosocial functioning throughout a patient's lifetime. PDs tend to remit slowly over time, but generally do not respond well to medication (Newton-Howes et al., 2006).

DIAGNOSING BORDERLINE PERSONALITY DISORDER

Borderline personality disorder (BPD) is a highly researched diagnosis, and there are thousands of papers about this condition in the literature. But it is not easy to treat, and it had, in the past, a reputation for incurability. Actually BPD has a fairly good prognosis, and we now have effective ways to treat many patients (Paris, 2010d). But I understand why clinicians want to avoid making the diagnosis. They see these patients as a source of endless trouble.

Since BPD is my sub-specialty and research interest, I am more concerned about underdiagnosis than overdiagnosis. However, overdiagnosis can occur—when every patient who cuts and overdoses is automatically considered to have the disorder. Overdiagnosis also occurs when clinicians jump to a diagnosis from one or two characteristic symptoms, and don't stop to count criteria. Not every patient who comes to the emergency room with a suicidal threat, an overdose, or self-harm has BPD.

With these problems in mind, I have chosen not to be satisfied with the overly broad definition of BPD offered in *DSM-5*. When you only need five of nine criteria, many permutations lead to the same diagnosis. Instead, I use a semi-structured interview (Diagnostic Interview for Border-lines, Revised, DIB-R; Zanarini et al., 1989) developed at McLean Hospital in Boston. This instrument narrows the range of patients who can meet criteria for the disorder. Unlike the *DSM*, it requires symptoms in multiple domains. Patients who meet the cutoff must also score at least 8/10 on the DIB-R, making it much more likely that they will fit a BPD prototype.

Underdiagnosis of BPD gives me concern because this is a serious mental disorder that requires specific treatment methods. Zimmerman et al. (2005) found that clinicians miss a *majority* of cases that meet criteria in structured interviews based on *DSM* criteria. Since patients with BPD often have a low mood, particularly when they come to an emergency room or a clinic, they often receive a diagnosis of major depression. They are usually prescribed antidepressants, even though the evidence for their effectiveness in this population is, as shown by a Cochrane report (Stoffers et al., 2012), rather poor.

When I was a resident, psychoanalysts on faculty encouraged me to diagnose BPD, because they believed that they had a treatment for it. But biological psychiatrists strongly discouraged me from believing that there was any such thing as BPD, because they preferred to concentrate on managing the depressive symptoms that accompany it. The situation has not entirely changed. BPD got a bad reputation because of its links to discredited theories of psychoanalysis. Some of the earlier definitions were based on obscure "metapsychological" processes that no one could measure. In a recent book, Michael Alan Taylor (2013), describing his long and profound distrust of psychoanalysis, rejected the BPD diagnosis, which he associated with that tradition. But Taylor sees *all* forms of psychotherapy as endless and fruitless talking. He wants to get on with "real" psychiatry, which involves writing the right prescription.

The most prominent expert to reject BPD is Hagop Akiskal, professor at the University of California, San Diego, and editor of the *Journal of Affective Disorders* (which he uses as a bully pulpit). One of his early articles (Akiskal et al., 1985) wittily described borderline as "an adjective without a noun." Ten years ago, I debated Akiskal about these issues in front of a large audience in Radio City Music Hall, at a New York meeting of the American Psychiatric Association—a story I have told in another book (Paris, 2012). Some people thought that I won that argument. But the misdiagnosis of PD as mood disorder is even more prevalent than it was then.

Akiskal had originally argued that BPD is a variant of depression. However, as Gunderson (2007) has noted, depression in BPD is phenomenologically distinct, with mood shifting mercurially within hours. Moreover, as confirmed by a Cochrane report (Stoffers et al., 2012), antidepressants are not very effective in BPD. (In spite of this research, nearly every patient is on them.) Akiskal (2002) later came to see BPD as a form of bipolarity. This view (discussed in Chapter 6) explains the affective instability and impulsivity that characterize BPD as a sub-clinical form of bipolar spectrum disorders.

A multi-center study of the boundaries of bipolarity, led by Jules Angst of Switzerland, a leading advocate of increased diagnosis, was recently published (Perugi et al., 2013), and suggested that BPD is overdiagnosed while bipolarity, broadly defined, is underdiagnosed. I was asked to contribute a commentary, and simply pointed out that phenomenology alone cannot determine the boundaries of mental disorders (Paris, 2013c). A second response, from a group that included the prominent Tufts University psychiatrist Nassir Ghaemi (Barroilhet et al., 2013) argued for the opposite conclusion. However, it was interesting that Barroilhet et al. thought it was sufficient to say that BPD was originally developed by psychoanalysts to determine that it must be invalid. Needless to say, these advocates entirely dismiss the published research on BPD.

Hostility toward the BPD diagnosis has done great harm to patients. Effective methods of psychotherapy are now available for this condition (Linehan, 1993; Bateman and Fonagy, 2004; Blum et al., 2008). Psychotherapy, when carefully designed and properly tested, is as scientific a method as any form of medication. But it no longer fits the spirit of the times, which favors a pharmacological fix.

OTHER PERSONALITY DISORDERS

DSM-5 lists 10 PDs, even though only two or three of them have been well researched. The others are a grab bag of dysfunctional traits and conditions, some of which border on serious mental illness. The hybrid proposal for *DSM-5* had quite rightly reduced the number of categories to six. As for the other four, to paraphrase Gilbert and Sullivan's *Mikado*, "there's none of them be missed."

Cluster A includes conditions that are close to schizophrenia. Schizotypal PD is cross-listed under the psychoses, as it is in *ICD-10*, and it is arguable that it does not really belong in PD but is closer to the schizophrenias (Siever, 2007). The difference is that schizotypal patients rarely develop frank psychosis. Patients with schizoid and paranoid

PD may also lie in the schizophrenic spectrum (Siever and Davis, 1991), but are even further from being frankly psychotic. The hybrid proposal would have folded these categories within schizotypal PD, and would have considered them as milder forms of the same disorder.

Cluster B includes ASPD and BPD, as well as two other categories. Histrionic PD is a diagnosis with an interesting history in psychiatry, as it used to be part of the now discredited concept of "hysteria" (Shorter, 1997). Today this category is rarely used, and was rightly slated for removal in the hybrid system.

Narcissistic personality disorder (NPD) was initially removed in the *DSM-5* proposals, but then (controversially) was reinstated. But reinstatement was the right decision. NPD is a good example of a pure trait disorder with few symptoms. For that reason, the large body of research on narcissistic traits (Campbell and Miller, 2011) is directly relevant to understanding patients who meet diagnostic criteria for this PD.

In Cluster C, we have avoidant PD, which is nearly identical to a category listed under anxiety disorders: social anxiety disorder. It has a very small research literature. We also have obsessive-compulsive PD, also poorly researched, as well as the category of dependent PD, which is vague and represents more of a trait than a mental disorder.

In summary, we have little reason to be concerned about the overdiagnosis of any PD category other than BPD. And that disorder is more likely to be missed entirely than to be wrongly diagnosed.

10

OTHER DISORDERS IN WHICH

OVERDIAGNOSIS IS A RISK

AUTISTIC SPECTRUM DISORDERS

Autism is a severe mental disorder that is poorly understood. There has long been little in the way of effective treatment, although that situation is beginning to change (Lai et al., 2013).

Given its severity, autism would not seem to be a likely candidate for overdiagnosis. Yet the prevalence of this condition in clinical settings and in epidemiological studies has gone up dramatically (Frances, 2013). Basu and Parry (2013) suggest that this increase (from two to five per 10,000 in 1960 to 50 to 114 per 10,000 in recent years) is the result of diagnostic "upcoding" whose real purpose is to justify the allocation of resources. The diagnostic epidemic of autism started quite a few years ago (Fombonne, 2001), and these issues remain controversial (Fombonne, 2009). We cannot be sure that the increase in the prevalence of the disorder is real.

Autism was first described 70 years ago by Kanner (1943), but was long considered rare. A primary feature of the classical disorder is its early onset, although children are normal until about age two, when symptoms first appear. In *DSM-IV*, milder conditions, including Asperger's syndrome, as well as pervasive developmental disorder, not otherwise specified (PDD-NOS), were added. In *DSM-5*, all of these diagnoses are classified as *autistic spectrum disorders*. This change was not based on the discovery of common biomarkers between diagnoses, but on phenomenological resemblances, which, much as in the bipolar spectrum, suggest a spectrum of severity. The problem lies in separating this spectrum from conditions that might have an entirely different etiology and pathogenesis.

There was some opposition to the new classification. It was not based on a lack of empirical support for the spectrum. Concern came from families who feared losing benefits for their children, particularly those diagnosed with Asperger's. From their point of view, they needed to be assured that children with milder cases would still be eligible for programs offering specialized care. A study comparing *DSM-IV* and *DSM-5* criteria (McPartlane et al., 2012) did find that fewer patients would qualify for an autistic spectrum diagnosis under the new system.

The idea that autism is a common disorder, not a rare one, is a dramatic change. A recent estimate of prevalence, based on parent reports, was 1% (Kogan et al., 2009), a much higher number than reported in the past. But it was trumped by a widely cited report from South Korea (Kim et al., 2011), estimating the community prevalence at 2.6%. That level would make autism nearly as common as major depression. The problem is that it is all too easy to categorize children who are shy or a bit peculiar as falling within the spectrum. These over-estimates of prevalence support the now common fear of parents that their children, if they deviate from what is perceived as a normal developmental path, could be autistic.

Patients who would have, in the past, been considered to meet criteria for other diagnoses, particularly intellectual deficiency, may now be receiving diagnoses of autism. Moreover, there could be an overlap with Cluster A personality disorders, in which people are notably strange without ever becoming psychotic. The diagnostic epidemic for autistic spectrum disorders may reflect a wish to develop broad concepts that provide a focus for research, which might eventually explain the origins of these puzzling disorders. While procedures have been suggested for the differential diagnosis of autism (Matson and Williams, 2013), there is no gold standard, so conclusions can only end up being a matter of clinical judgment.

The increase in the prevalence of autism began before there was much treatment, but recent evidence suggests that intensive therapies can be effective, at least to some extent (Thompson, 2013). These findings require replication, and we know from experience with other brain disorders (such as schizophrenia) that results can be incomplete and slow in coming. Yet families generally insist on these treatments, which are lengthy and very expensive. This is the driving force that will probably continue the current pattern of overdiagnosis.

ANXIETY DISORDERS

Horwitz and Wakefield (2012) pointed out that psychiatry views anxiety as more of a clinical problem than a normal response to life's dangers. As we saw in Chapter 7, PTSD has been a particular target for overdiagnosis. Similar trends can be seen, however, for generalized anxiety disorder (GAD). This was a new diagnosis in *DSM-III*, separated from panic disorder by the absence of discrete episodes. It describes patients who worry too much, have physical symptoms of anxiety, and who are chronically anxious rather than suffering from panic attacks. Because GAD is a catch-all, the diagnosis is popular.

GAD has a moderately high prevalence of 1.5% (Kessler et al., 2005a), but more people have sub-clinical symptoms. Clinical cases of GAD may overlap with depression, and when both are diagnosed, the clinical picture is more severe (Zimmerman and Chelminski, 2003). The *DSM-5* process originally proposed widening the criteria for GAD, but in the end, they were left unchanged (Starkevic and Portman, 2013).

Another diagnosis of concern for overdiagnosis is social anxiety disorder, which is difficult to separate from extreme shyness (Lane, 2007; Horwitz and Wakefield, 2012). The community prevalence of this condition suggests that it is common, with estimates ranging from 4% to as high as 13% (Wittchen and Fehm, 2001). This immediately raises questions. Is the condition defined in a way that makes overdiagnosis easy? Have the drug companies promoted this diagnosis to raise sales of antidepressants (Lane, 2007)? Of is this just another example of the medicalization of variant traits?

REVISING OLD CATEGORIES AND CREATING NEW ONES

The *DSM* system has widened the criteria for some diagnoses, and has also created diagnoses that are either new or that offer a relabeling of old categories. It is hard to predict which of these will lead to diagnostic epidemics. Frances (2013) warns of this possibility, but we have no data on most changes—either of innovations or of revised criteria.

However, history suggests that something of this nature is likely to happen. Inflated prevalence followed from the introduction of bipolar-II and adult ADHD in *DSM-IV*. Similar effects could be seen for the newer categories in *DSM-5*.

Consider, for example, *mild neurocognitive disorder*, whose introduction was the major change in this section of the manual (Blazer, 2013). The category describes changes in cognitive function that could be early signs of dementia, but could also represent little more than the normative decline that all people experience as they age. We do not know whether this condition will be overdiagnosed, but since many people today worry about developing major neurocognitive disorders such as Alzheimer's, it is a distinct possibility.

Similar problems could arise from a few diagnoses that were promoted from the Appendix of *DSM-IV* to the main body of *DSM-5*. One was *binge eating disorder*. Again, the problem is whether behavior that is highly prevalent in the general population is a diagnosis that could be applied to normal people. An international survey, the World Health Organization (WHO) World Mental Health Surveys (Kessler et al., 2013), found a median prevalence of 1%, higher than bulimia nervosa. While the authors expressed concern about a largely untreated public health issue, the high number may only reflect the broad definition of disorder that was adopted. In any case, binge eating is a symptom that can be seen in many other conditions.

Another promotion from the Appendix to the main section was *premenstrual dysphoric disorder*. This diagnosis has been controversial because it medicalizes phenomena that are common in normal women. Epperson et al. (2012), reviewing data for including it in the new edition, estimated its prevalence at 2%–4%. Whether or not this decision will lead to inflated prevalence in clinical populations is unknown. Even without approval from the *DSM*, this syndrome has often been treated with antidepressants.

Each of these changes had its proponents, and each had a constituency of researchers and sub-specialists convinced that the conditions that interested them were either under-recognized or needed a more inclusive definition. Needless to say, no one thinks of cost-benefit when revising a diagnostic manual. With the best of intentions, we could be in for more cases of inflated prevalence and diagnostic epidemics in the coming years.

PART THREE

DIAGNOSIS AND NORMALITY

11

HOW DO WE KNOW

WHAT IS NORMAL?

NORMALITY AND MEDICINE

To determine what is pathological, you must define what is normal. This task is not simple. If you look hard enough, most people live in a delicate balance between sickness and health. For that reason, no one is normal in every way and at all times. Most people live with some degree of distress. But when researchers carry out screening procedures in non-clinical populations, many people who are not symptomatic will nonetheless be diagnosed. Positive screening does not equal diagnosis.

In medicine, we sometimes treat the common cold, and we might do so more often if we had an effective treatment. In this framework, one can understand why patients with the mildest symptoms can still receive a diagnosis. Organs do not function perfectly, and there is no definite point at which biomarkers that deviate from a norm can be considered abnormal. For example, elevations of blood sugar or cholesterol in people who do not have symptoms may or may not be signs of illness. You can only call laboratory findings pathological if they are associated with the clinical features of disease, or will eventually lead to disease.

These problems are not particular to psychiatry. Welch et al. (2011) have described the extent to which overdiagnosis (and over-investigation to look for diagnoses) has become a conundrum in medical practice. One reason is that physicians are trained to look for pathology, and above all, not to *miss* anything. Patients may also insist on blood tests and scans to produce a diagnosis that will explain why they are suffering.

At the extreme, the presence of illness is usually clear. A very high glucose level will usually be the result of diabetes. But definitions of cutoff points can change over time, so that even minor variations may become considered as clinical problems requiring treatment. Yet people can have changes, such as an elevated cholesterol level, without falling ill, or even being at significant risk for being ill.

In the past, patients went to doctors when they had symptoms, but they did not necessarily expect a diagnosis. Today, influenced by the media, they are more likely to seek a label that explains symptoms. Moreover, physicians are trained to investigate patients aggressively, using tools such as imaging that gather much more information. The result is that unimportant abnormalities are identified, leading to even further investigations. In the world of scanning, radiologists call such non-meaningful findings "incidentomas" (Welch et al., 2011).

Many findings that are observed only through investigative procedures, and that do not produce symptoms, can be noted but safely ignored. A good example is prostate cancer in situ (Djulbegovic et al., 2010). By a certain age, about half of all men will have carcinoma cells somewhere in their prostate gland. But in the vast majority of cases, clinical symptoms do not develop, and patients eventually die of something else. Another example is mammography, which the Cochrane Collaboration (Gøtzsche and Nielsen, 2011) considers to be doubtfully effective for preventing breast cancer. It has even been suggested that cancer screening can do more harm than good (Esserman et al., 2013).

NORMALITY IN PSYCHIATRY

In psychiatry, normality is defined behaviorally, rather than on the basis of biomarkers. In some ways, this might be a good thing—we don't have to worry, at least for now, that a blood test or a scan will be used to support the overdiagnosis of mental illness. However, naïve faith in structured clinical assessments, screening procedures, and psychological testing are creating much the same problem.

Epidemiological research (Kessler et al., 2005b) has led many to the conclusion that mental illness of one kind or another is ubiquitous. The idea is that subclinical forms of disorder are common and untreated. For example, Van Os (2009), a researcher on schizophrenia, argues that mental disorders have "sub-threshold extended phenotypes," which are nonspecific and indistinct, but that constitute risk factors for diagnosable disorders. Even if that conclusion is correct, it does not follow that we should aggressively promote prevention and early intervention in people who may be at risk, but who will, in most cases, never develop severe mental disorders. To determine whether such programs are truly effective, we would need the kind of solid evidence that we have for links between smoking and cancer. In the absence of such evidence, it makes more sense to concentrate our limited resources on patients who are more obviously ill, not on those who have risk factors or are living with subclinical symptoms. Mental health professionals, who have sick patients to look after, have better things to do than screening normal people.

McGorry et al. (2008) state that while there can be problems with both over-treatment and under-treatment, when symptoms are persistent and severe, we do the population a disservice by failing to intervene. The focus is on identifying and treating risk psychosis, which might be used to prevent chronicity. But this diagnosis, suggested for *DSM-5*, was not included because of a high rate of false positives (Morrison et al., 2012). Similarly, screening for depression identifies many people who do not need to be treated (Thombs et al., 2008). And since there is a significant risk associated with prescribing antidepressants, one should not rush to intervention without good evidence that doing so is cost-effective.

For all the effort that has gone into screening and early detection of illness in medicine, the value of doing so has not been well established. Well-meaning attempts at prevention may actually do harm to people by offering them treatments they do not need, and that have side effects of their own. What we call "normal" in medicine can include phenomena that interfere with ideal functioning, but have no practical significance. If physicians treat every variation in traits or symptoms as pathological, patients will not be well served.

Welch et al. (2011) emphasize the importance of distinguishing between early diagnosis and population screening. If we knew for sure who is at high risk, there would be nothing wrong with identifying such cases and treating them early. But we don't know. The best example would be the prescription of antipsychotics to people with risk psychosis, 70% of whom will never develop schizophrenia, and who would be harmed rather than benefited by treatment. Another is the prescription of antidepressants to patients who are not clinically depressed (Mojtabai, 2013). That practice fails to recognize that sadness is part of the human condition.

Psychiatry's enthusiasm for early identification of illness, and for screening in the community, runs parallel to developments in medicine as a whole. The problem is to set thresholds that are clinically meaningful. Just as most people can have a few abnormal laboratory findings or incidentomas, everyone experiences some degree of psychological distress and/or dysfunction, at least from time to time. The challenges of modern life mean that people are not always successful at managing work tasks and/or intimate relationships. When people lose their jobs or their partners, they will probably be sad. To call this depression is to pathologize normality.

Overdiagnosis, in both psychiatry and medicine, leads to over-treatment, which may not be benign. If unhappy people are seen as depressed, they can be prescribed medications for years on end that carry significant side effects, or can spend years of their life attending psychotherapy sessions that provide little more than support.

All these trends reflect a deeper cultural change: the wish to be "better than well" (Elliott, 2003). Perhaps people in the past had lower expectations, and were more stoical about life's vicissitudes. Today, we expect health, happiness, and "self-realization." Wanting perfection, we have forgotten what is normal.

In his book *Saving Normal*, Allen Frances (2013) criticizes *DSM-5* for encouraging a diagnostic expansion that leaves little room for the concept of normality. Frances is right, but the problem does not lie with the manual. It derives from a medical culture that promotes overdiagnosis, and from cultural expectations that the health professions should provide an answer to every life problem. Nor is the problem entirely new—psychoanalysis, like today's biological psychiatry, long claimed that it could make normal people better than well.

DEFINITIONS OF NORMALITY

Diagnosis in psychiatry suffers from its inability to define what is normal. *DSM-5* attempts to define mental disorder (not very successfully), but is silent on the subject of normality. Attempts to produce a valid definition go back many decades (Offer and Sabshin, 1966).

One definition is that normality represents an average, so that deviations from a mean score on any measure determine what is abnormal. However, this approach suffers from serious problems. In societies where disease is rampant (tuberculosis in nineteenth-century Europe, malaria in contemporary Africa), what is average may not be at all normal. Also, at what cutoff point does deviation from the mean imply pathology? Internists face this problem every day in evaluating at what point an increase in blood pressure constitutes illness. Similarly, psychiatrists have to determine whether painful emotions such as depression or anxiety constitute mental disorders. Finally, psychological experiences are influenced by social norms, so that what is pathological in one society could be normal in another. The *DSM* consistently fails to separate responses that are understandable in a social context from psychopathology that is intrinsic to the individual and relatively context-independent (Horwitz and Wakefield, 2007).

A second approach to normality is to define it in terms of function versus dysfunction. Wakefield's (1992) concept of mental disorder as "harmful dysfunction" depends on the assumption that we can know what is functional, by establishing whether psychological states are or are not performing a purpose related to the demands of natural selection. Yet this determination is not as easy as it sounds, since functionality lies on a continuum. If there is no clear break between function and dysfunction, then deciding what is and what is not illness remains a judgment call. In any case, the demands of living in the modern world no longer retain a close correspondence to biological evolution. That is one reason that homosexuality is no longer considered to be a mental disorder.

In summary, neither a statistical nor a functional definition allows for a reliable definition of normality. Our inability to make these distinctions makes clinical judgment the ultimate arbiter.

Life can be a bumpy road, and we should not expect to be consistently happy. The rise of overdiagnosis in psychiatry has obscured a basic truth about the medicalization of suffering. If, as epidemiological research suggests, most people meet criteria for at least one category of disorder as defined by the *DSM* across their lifetime, there may be something over-inclusive about our definition of illness. We should consider that lower levels of symptoms can be normal reactions to circumstance. It would probably be better to define mental health, not as happiness, but as resilience in the face of adversity. This is not to say that extreme circumstances cannot cause mental disorders—they can. But we do not need to pathologize the human condition.

MEDICALIZATION, OVERDIAGNOSIS, AND SOCIAL STRESSORS

One consequence of medicalization and overdiagnosis is the failure to identify social stressors that produce psychological distress (Horwitz, 2007). Diagnosis inevitably places the locus of pathology in the individual, and not in the social circumstances in which we live. Instead of identifying social stressors (some of which might be remediable), psychiatry overestimates the number of people who have mental disorders and promotes "unmet needs" for treatment.

The current focus of psychiatry on neurobiology downplays the role of psychosocial stressors. In the most validated disorders, research shows that the failure to find effective social roles is a risk factor, even for psychosis (Dutta and Murray, 2010), and that suicide is more likely to occur under conditions of alienation and weak attachment (Durkheim, 1897/1951). Stressful conditions may be of even greater importance for people who are normal but unhappy. For example, low socioeconomic status has been consistently shown to increase distress (Eaton and Muntaner, 1999). While social stressors are risk factors for mental disorders, to qualify for a diagnosis, the response of the individual must be excessive and out of proportion, reflecting either biological or psychological fragility. The problem with the overdiagnosis that has been supported by the *DSM* system is that this distinction is lost—*anyone* with a sufficient level of symptoms can be categorized as having a disorder, whether the response is deemed to be proportionate or disproportionate (Horwitz, 2007).

Medicalization of psychological distress is also promoted by the ready availability of screening tools on the Internet. I can hardly count the number of patients who have told me they have bipolar disorder or ADHD after scoring themselves on one of these instruments. Further confirmation can come from tools provided by the pharmaceutical industry, or by mental health advocacy groups. And physicians, anxious to be helpful, are often ready to confirm these impressions by treating patients for these conditions.

HOW THE LOSS OF NORMAL DOES HARM

Horwitz (2007) acknowledges the good intentions behind the medicalization of distress. But, as Frances (2013) points out, instead of reducing stigma, diagnosis, if inaccurate, can unnecessarily increase it. I have a different concern: that over-treatment usually follows overdiagnosis.

In the heyday of psychoanalysis, everyone was advised to lie on a couch and explore their psyche, whether or not they had a mental disorder. Actually taking that path did minimal harm, except for the enormous waste of time and money on a procedure of dubious value. The situation is quite different when the treatment for unhappiness consists of medication. Fortunately, antidepressants are relatively harmless, and people can take them for years (as they now often do) without suffering serious side effects. This is not the case for antipsychotics. Physicians have the impression that second-generation drugs do not produce severe problems, but they often do. We do not know the long-term outcome of prescribing them over years to patients with anxiety or depression.

In 2013, the American Psychiatric Association joined the "Choosing Wisely" Campaign, sponsored by organized medicine in the United States. This initiative attempts to set better guidelines for treatment in all medical specialties. Psychiatry has made firm recommendations about limiting the use of antipsychotic drugs: that they should not be used as a first-line intervention in non-psychotic disorders, or for insomnia that can be managed in other ways (www.psychiatry. org/13-58-Choosing-Wisely-announcement.pdf). One can only hope that psychiatrists are listening to their own organization, and not to the incessant propaganda put out by Big Pharma.

Medicine must be based on scientific evidence, even if practicing in that way sometimes displeases patients. We need to be much more cautious about moving to a prescribing mode. We also need to tell patients when they are going though a normal "bad patch." This need not be a dismissal of suffering, since it is entirely legitimate to see a therapist when going through a difficult time. But when assessment produces a diagnostic label that patients can carry with them for years, and when it leads to an unnecessary drug prescription that also goes on for years, it does more harm than good.

Ultimately, the concept of normality is a philosophical issue. If you think life should be "better than well," you will seek to fix every problem by considering it to be a treatable medical condition. If, on the other hand, you accept that life is difficult at best, and that living presents continuous challenges, you are more likely to accept life's inevitable vicissitudes. This is not to say that we should passively accept unnecessary suffering, or that medicine has not contributed an enormous amount to the length and quality of all our lives. But overdiagnosis, cutting across normality, over-stretches these principles to a breaking point. Life does not need to be perfect, or even consistently happy, but just good enough to make it worthwhile.

12

WHERE DO WE GO FROM HERE?

OVERDIAGNOSIS AND UNCERTAINTY

Physicians are not the only ones responsible for overdiagnosis. But they could put a stop to it if they chose to. Intolerance for uncertainty tempts us to come up with easy answers to hard questions.

Who are the other players? The media have played a role in overdiagnosis. Reporters are always looking for a story, and the idea that one disorder or another is producing terrible suffering, while being under-recognized, seems to be irresistible. Finally, the pharmaceutical industry, which obtained direct access to the public for advertising in the United States, has played a key role, feeding on the public perception that doctors always understand disease, and that there are effective drugs for every symptom.

Patients and their families have played a crucial role. We live in an age of consumerism, a movement that has affected the way in which medicine is practiced. Patients are no longer passive recipients of treatment, or totally in awe of medical authority. Many come armed with their own literature searches, and want to participate in decisions. Advocacy groups have sprung up to defend the interests of patients and their families. For this reason, ironically, diagnostic epidemics can be supported by the people who suffer from them.

By and large, consumerism in medicine is a good thing. But patients are susceptible to accept false beliefs about the diagnosis and treatment of mental disorders. The problem may not be recognized, because patients who see things the same way as their mental health providers will find few reasons to complain.

The positive side of consumerism is that every patient has a right to know his or her diagnosis. But that does not mean that information should be communicated dogmatically. Practitioners, once they are aware of the uncertainty around diagnosis, could feel comfortable with saying something like "your problems are most consistent with diagnosis X, and we will treat you for that, but since we can't be sure, let's keep our minds open."

I was surprised to find that sharing information with patients can still be controversial. A debate in the *British Medical Journal* (Callard et al., 2013) examined whether patients in the mental health system actually benefit from being told what the physician thinks is wrong with them. But this debate failed to ask a crucial question—how do we know that a diagnosis is right? Perhaps to admit that psychiatric diagnosis is inexact is a way of saying that the emperor has no clothes.

One can understand why patients search so hard for explanations, and why they become so attached to categories of disorder. When a diagnosis is known to be valid and guides the choice of effective treatment, the process is positive. But when it simply labels symptoms and leads to treatment that is of doubtful value, the process is negative.

Almost every day, I hear patients tell me that they (or a relative) have been diagnosed with a disorder, usually on the basis of a few clinical symptoms and/or a nonspecific testing procedure. What this tells us is that physicians, like most people, avoid doubt and are attracted to certainty. But when it comes to identifying the nature of a mental disorder, doubt is the only place to start.

OVERCOMING OVERDIAGNOSIS

Evidence-based practice is now widely accepted as a guiding principle in medicine and psychiatry. It has been an enormous force for good. We should continue to encourage physicians and their patients to rely on data rather than on clinical experience or opinion. But when you study the scientific literature carefully, you often come up with more questions than answers. Since most research findings in medicine turn out to be non-replicable (Ioannidis, 2005), you have to wait for meta-analyses and Cochrane reports to be sure that any conclusion is correct, or to be sure that any treatment is effective. Depending on softer indices of outcome is treacherous. For example, you cannot depend on indications for pharmaceutical agents that are approved by the Food and Drug Administration: they only require two trials, usually funded by industry. The best attitude for a practicing physician is a reasonable level of optimism, strongly tempered by caution and skepticism.

In the same way, psychiatry should adopt *evidence-based diagnosis*. Doing so would subject the diagnostic process to the same caution and skepticism as have been applied to the results of treatment research. We can view new diagnoses, or wider applications of old diagnoses, with interest, but wait patiently to see how they pan out. The main antidote for overdiagnosis is to avoid unnecessary enthusiasm. Fads and epidemics are driven by the need for certainty (Paris, 2013b). What we might do better to cultivate is uncertainty.

This requires taking a long view. Diagnoses come and go, and not all have remained stable since the introduction of systematic classification. When I was a student, we were taught *DSM-I*. In 50 years, *DSM-5* will also be seen as a historical curiosity. Psychiatrists of the future will wonder how those who practiced in the early twenty-first century could have been so naïve as to take these categories so seriously.

I feel optimistic that in the long run, the level of overdiagnosis we see today will become an amusing historical curiosity. When we know more, we will have less reason to over-simplify clinical problems. The diagnostic manuals of the future will probably not look very much like *DSM-5*. Nor will they resemble the RDoC system. I expect that they will be based on a deeper and more thorough understanding of disease. But that will take many decades, and we have to remain humble and patient.

This book has advocated humility in the face of ignorance. It has also argued that psychiatrists have little to be ashamed of. We are at the very beginning of a long journey that will lead us into an unimaginable future. Overdiagnosis creates the illusion that we already know the answers. We must have the courage to admit that, at this point, we don't.

REFERENCES

Abrams, R, Taylor, MA. (1981): Importance of schizophrenic symptoms in the diagnosis of mania. *American Journal of Psychiatry*, 138: 658–661.

Addington, J, Epstein, I, Reynolds, A, Furimsky, I, Rudy, L, Mancini, B, et al. (2008): Early detection of psychosis: finding those at clinical high risk, *Early Intervention in Psychiatry*, 2: 147–153.

Akiskal HS, Chen SE, Davis GC. (1985): Borderline: an adjective in search of a noun. *Journal of Clinical Psychiatry*, 46: 41–48.

Akiskal, HS. (2002): The bipolar spectrum: the shaping of a new paradigm in psychiatry. *Current Psychiatry Reports*, 4: 1–3.

Akiskal, HS, Akiskal, KK, Lancrenon, S, Hantouche, EG, Fraud, J-P, Gury, C, et al. (2006): Validating the bipolar spectrum in the French National EPIDEP Study: overview of the phenomenology and relative prevalence of its clinical prototypes. *Journal of Affective Disorders*, 96: 197–205.

Akiskal, HS, McKinney, WT, Jr. (1973): Depressive disorders: toward a unified hypothesis, *Science*, 182: 20–29.

Altman, DG, Bland, JM. (1994): Diagnostic tests: sensitivity and specificity. *BMJ*, 308 (6943): 1552.

American Psychiatric Association. (2010). *Practice Guideline for the Treatment of Patients with Major Depressive Disorder* (2nd ed.). Washington, DC: American Psychiatric Press.

American Psychiatric Association. (2013): *Diagnostic and Statistical Manual of Mental Disorders* (5th ed.). Washington, DC: Author.

Angell, M. (2000): Is academic medicine for sale? *New England Journal of Medicine*, 342: 1516–1518.

Angold, A, Erkanli, A, Egger, HL, Costello, EJ. (2000): Stimulant treatment for children: a community perspective. *Journal of the American Academy of Child & Adolescent Psychiatry*, 39: 975–984.

Baer, RA, Peters, JR, Eisenhlorh, TA, Geiger, PJ, Sauer, SE. (2012): Emotion-related cognitive processes in borderline personality disorder: a review of the empirical literature. *Clinical Psychology Review*, 32: 359–369.

Barkley, RA. (2006): *Attention–Deficit Hyperactivity Disorder: A Handbook For Diagnosis and Treatment* (3rd ed.). New York: Guilford Press.

Barroilhet, S, Vohringer, PA, Ghaemi, SN. (2013): Borderline versus bipolar: differences matter. *Acta Psychiatrica Scandinavica* 128: 385–386.

Basu, S, Parry, P. (2013): The autism spectrum disorder 'epidemic': need for biopsychosocial formulation. *Australian and New Zealand Journal of Psychiatry* (in press), 47: 1116–1118.

Bateman, A, Fonagy, P. (2004): *Psychotherapy for Borderline Personality Disorder: Mentalization Based Treatment*. Oxford: Oxford University Press.

Batstra, L, Frances, AJ. (2012): DSM-5 further inflates Attention Deficit Hyperactivity Disorder. *Journal of Nervous and Mental Diseases*, 200: 486–488.

Beck, AT. (2008): The evolution of the cognitive model of depression and its neurobiological correlates. *American Journal of Psychiatry*, 165: 969–977.

Biederman J, Newcorn, J, Sprich, S. (1991): Comorbidity of attention deficit hyperactivity disorder with conduct, depressive, anxiety, and other disorders. *American Journal of Psychiatry*, 148: 564–577.

Bishop, D, Rutter, M. (2009): Neurodevelopmental disorders: conceptual issues. In Rutter, M, Bishop, DVM, Pine, DS, Scott, S, Stevenson, J, Taylor E, Thapar, A (Eds.), *Rutter's Child and Adolescent Psychiatry* (5th ed.) Oxford: Blackwell Publishing.

Biskin, R, Paris, J. (2012): Diagnosis of borderline personality disorder. *Canadian Medical Association Journal*, 184: 1789–1794.

Black, DW, Gunter, T, Loveless, P, Allen, J. (2010): Antisocial personality disorder in incarcerated offenders: Psychiatric comorbidity and quality of life. *Annals of Clinical Psychiatry*, 22: 113–120.

Black, DW, Grant, JE. (2014): *DSM-5 Guidebook: The Essential Companion to the Diagnostic and Statistical Manual of Mental Disorders, Fifth Edition.* Washington, DC: American Psychiatric Publishing.

Blazer, D. (2013): Neurocognitive disorders in DSM-5. *American Journal of Psychiatry*, 170: 585–587.

Blier, P. (2008): Do antidepressants really work? *Journal of Psychiatry & Neuroscience*, 33: 89–90.

Bloom, P. (2004): *Descartes' Baby: How the Science of Child Development Explains What Makes Us Human.* New York: Basic Books.

Blum, N, St John, D, Pfohl, B, Black, DW. (2008): Systems Training for Emotional Predictability and Problem Solving (STEPPS) for outpatients with borderline personality disorder: a randomized controlled trial and 1-year follow-up. *American Journal of Psychiatry*, 165: 468–478.

Bosanac, P, Patton, GC, Castle, DJ. (2010): Early intervention in psychotic disorders: faith before facts. *Psychological Medicine*, 40(3): 353–358.

Bracken, P, Thomas, P, Timimi, S, Asen, E. (2012): Psychiatry beyond the current paradigm. *British Journal of Psychiatry*, 201: 430–434.

Brady, K, Pearlstein, T, Asnis, GM, Baker, D, Rothbaum, B, Sikes, CR, Farfel, GM. (2000): Efficacy and safety of sertraline treatment of posttraumatic stress disorder: a randomized controlled trial. *Journal of the American Medical Association*, 283: 1837–1844.

Breslau, N, Davis, GC, Andreski, P (1991): Traumatic events and posttraumatic stress disorder in an urban population of young adults. *Archives of General Psychiatry*, 48: 216–222.

Breslau, N, Bohnert, KM, Koenen, KC. (2010): The 9/11 attack and post-traumatic stress disorder revisited. *Journal of Nervous & Mental Disease*, 198: 539–543.

Cade, JF. (1949): Lithium salts in the treatment of psychotic excitement. *Medical Journal of Australia*, 3: 349–352.

Callard, F, Bracken, P, David, P, Sarotrius, N. (2013): Has psychiatric diagnosis labelled rather than enabled patients? *BMJ*, 347: f4312.

Campbell, WK, Miller, JD. (2011): *Handbook of Narcissism and Narcissistic Personality Disorder*. New York: Wiley.

Casacalenda, N, Boulenger, JP. (1998): Pharmacological treatments effective in both generalized anxiety disorder and major depressive disorder: clinical and theoretical implications. *Canadian Journal of Psychiatry*, 43: 722–730.

Centers for Disease Control. (2011): Prevalence of attention-deficit hyperactivity disorder. http://www.cdc.gov/ncbddd/adhd/prevalence.html, accessed October 2013.

Chan, D, Sireling, L. (2010): "I want to be bipolar". . . a new phenomenon. *The Psychiatrist*, 34: 103–105.

Cipriani, AA, Furukawa, TA, Salanti, G, Geddes, JR, Higgins, JPT, Churchill, R, Watanabe, N, Nakagawa, A, Omori, IM, McGuire, H, Tansella, M, Barbui, C. (2009): Comparative efficacy and acceptability of 12 new-generation antidepressants: a multiple-treatments meta-analysis. *Lancet*, 373: 746–758.

Coid, J, Yang, M, Tyrer, P, Roberts, A, Ullrich, S. (2006): Prevalence and correlates of personality disorder in Great Britain. *British Journal of Psychiatry*, 188: 423–431.

Comer, JS, Mojtabai, R, Olfson, M. (2011): National trends in the antipsychotic treatment of psychiatric outpatients with anxiety disorders. *American Journal of Psychiatry*, 168: 1057–1065.

Cooper, JE, Kendell, RE, Gurland, BJ. (1972): *Psychiatric Diagnosis in New York and London*. London: Oxford University Press.

Corrigan, PW, ed. (2005): *On the Stigma of Mental Illness: Practical Strategies for Research and Social Change*. Washington, DC: American Psychological Association.

Costa, PT, Widiger, TA (Eds.). (2013): *Personality Disorders and the Five Factor Model of Personality* (3rd ed.). Washington, DC: American Psychological Association.

Craddock, N, Owen, MJ. (2005): The beginning of the end for the Kraepelinian dichotomy. *British Journal of Psychiatry*, 186: 364–366.

Cronbach, LJ, Meehl, PE. (1951): Construct validity in psychological tests. *Psychological Bulletin*, 52: 281–302.

Cukor, J, Spitalnick, Difede, J, Rizzo, A, Rothbaum, BO. (2009): Emerging treatments for PTSD. *Clinical Psychology Review*, 29: 715–726.

Cumyn, L, French, L, Hechtman L. (2009): Comorbidity in adults with attention-deficit hyperactivity disorder. *Canadian Journal of Psychiatry*, 54: 673–683.

Danaei, G, Ding, EL, Mozaffarian, D, Taylor, B, Rehhm, J, Murray, C, Ezzati, M. (2009): The preventable causes of death in the United States: comparative risk assessment of dietary, lifestyle, and metabolic risk factors. *PLOS Medicine* 6(4): e1000058. doi:10.1371/journal.pmed.1000058.

Decker, H. (2013): *Making the DSM-III*. New York: Oxford University Press.

deRaedt, R, Koster, EHW. (2010): Understanding vulnerability for depression from a cognitive neuroscience perspective: a reappraisal of attentional factors and a new conceptual framework. *Cognitive, Affective, & Behavioral Neuroscience*, 10: 50–70.

Djulbegovic, M, Beyth, RJ, Dahm, P. (2010): Screening for prostate cancer: systematic review and meta-analysis of randomised controlled trials. *British Medical Journal*, 341: 4543

Dunner, DI, Tay, KL. (1993): Diagnostic reliability of the history of hypomania in bipolar II patients and patients with major depression. *Comprehensive Psychiatry*, 34: 303–307.

Durkheim, E. (1897/1951). *Suicide: A Study in Sociology*. New York: Free Press.

Durston, S. (2003): A review of the biological bases of ADHD: what have we learned from imaging studies? *Mental Retardation and Developmental Disabilities Research Reviews*, 9: 184–195.

Dutta, R, Murray, RM. (2010): A life-course approach to psychosis: outcome and cultural variation. In Millon, T, Krueger, R, Simonsen, E. (Eds.), *Contemporary Directions in Psychopathology: Scientific Foundations of the DSM-V and ICD 11.* New York: Guilford Press, pp. 515–522.

Eaton, WW, Muntaner, C. (1999): Socioeconomic stratification and mental disorder. In Horwitz, AV, Scheid, TA (Eds.), *A Handbook for the Study of Mental Health: Social Contexts,*

Theories, and Systems. New York: Cambridge University Press, pp. 259–283.

Eisenberg, L. (1986): Mindlessness and brainlessness in psychiatry. *British Journal of Psychiatry*, 148: 497–508.

Elliott, C. (2003): *Better Than Well: American Medicine Meets the American Dream*. New York: Norton.

Engel, GL. (1980): The clinical application of the biopsychosocial model. *American Journal of Psychiatry*, 137: 535–544.

Epperson, CN, Steiner, M, Yonkers, KA. (2012): Premenstrual dysphoric disorder: evidence for a new category for DSM-5. *American Journal of Psychiatry*, 169: 465–475.

Esserman, LJ, Thompson, IM, Reid, B. (2013): Overdiagnosis and overtreatment in cancer: an opportunity for improvement. *Journal of the American Medical Association*, 310: 797–798.

Faraone, SV, Sergeant, J, Gillberg, C, Biederman, J. (2000): The worldwide prevalence of attention deficit hyperactivity disorder. *Journal of the American Academy of Child & Adolescent Psychiatry*, 39: 182–193.

Faraone, SV, Sergeant, J, Gillberg, C. (2003): The worldwide prevalence of ADHD: is it an American disorder? *World Psychiatry*, 2: 104–113.

Faraone, SV. (2005): The scientific foundation for understanding attention deficit/hyperactivity disorder as a valid psychiatric disorder. *European Journal of Child and Adolescent Psychiatry*, 14: 1–10.

First, MB. (2011): DSM-5 proposals for mood disorders: a cost–benefit analysis. *Current Opinion in Psychiatry*, 24: 1–9.

Fombonne, E. (2001): Is there an epidemic of autism? *Pediatrics*, 107: 411–412.

Fombonne, E. (2009): Epidemiology of pervasive developmental disorders. *Pediatric Research*, 65: 591–598.

Fournier, JC, DeRubeis, RJ, Hollon, SD, Dimidjian, S, Amsterdam, JD, Shelton, R, Fawcett, J. (2010): Antidepressant drug effects and depression severity: a patient-level meta-analysis. *Journal of the American Medical Association*, 303: 47–53.

Frances, A. (2013): *Saving Normal*. New York: Morrow.

Frank, JD, Frank, JB. (1991): *Persuasion and Healing* (3rd ed.). Baltimore, MD: Johns Hopkins.

Fulford, KWM, Thornton, T, Graham, G (Eds.). (2006). *Oxford Textbook of Philosophy and Psychiatry*. New York: Oxford University Press.

Furedi, F. (2003): *Therapy Culture*. New York: Routledge.

Geddes, JR, for the **BALANCE investigators and collaborators** (2010): Lithium plus valproate combination therapy versus monotherapy for relapse prevention in bipolar I disorder (BALANCE): a randomised open-label trial. *Lancet*, 375: 35–352.

Gold, I. (2009): Reduction in psychiatry. *Canadian Journal of Psychiatry*, 54: 506–512.

Goodwin, FK, Jamison, K. (2007): *Manic-Depressive Illness: Bipolar Disorder and Recurrent Depression* (2nd ed.). New York: Oxford University Press.

Gordon, T. (2000): *Parent Effectiveness Training: The Proven Program for Raising Responsible Children*. New York: Random House.

Gøtzsche, PC, Nielsen, M. (2011): Screening for breast cancer with mammography. *Cochrane Database Syst Rev* (1): CD001877. doi:10.1002/14651858.CD001877.pub4. PMID 21249649.

Greenberg, G. (2013): *The Book of Woe*. New York: Penguin.

Gunderson, JG. (2013): DSM-5: Current status, lessons learned, and future challenges. *Personality Disorders: Theory, Research, Treatment*, 4: 378–380.

Gunderson, JG, Weinberg, I, Daversa, M, Kueppenbender, KD, Zanarini, MC, Shea, MT, Skodol, AE, Sanislow, CA, Yen, S, Morey, LC, Grilo, CM, McGlashan, TH, Stout, RL, Dyck, I. (2006): Descriptive and longitudinal observations on the relationship of borderline personality disorder and bipolar disorder. *American Journal of Psychiatry*, 163: 1173–1178.

Hamilton, M. (1959): The assessment of anxiety states by rating. *British Journal of Medical Psychology*, 32: 50–55.

Hansen, R, Gaynes, B, Thieda, P, Gartlehner, G, Deveaugh-Geiss, A, Krebs, E, Lohr, K (2008): Meta-analysis of major depressive disorder relapse and recurrence with second-generation antidepressants *Psychiatric Services*, 59: 1121–1130.

Hirschfeld, RMA. (2000): Antidepressants in long-term therapy: a review of tricyclic antidepressants and selective serotonin reuptake inhibitors. *Acta Psychiatrica Scandinavica*, 101(S403): 35–38.

Hoch, PH, Cattell, JP, Strahl, MD, Penness, HH. (1962). The course and outcome of pseudoneurotic schizophrenia. *American Journal of Psychiatry*, 119: 106–115.

Horwitz, AV. (2007): Transforming normality into pathology: the *DSM* and the outcomes of stressful social arrangements. *Journal of Health and Social Behavior*, 48: 211–219.

Horwitz, AV, Wakefield, JC. (2007): *The Loss of Sadness: How Psychiatry Transformed Normal Sorrow Into Depressive Disorder*. New York: Oxford University Press.

Horwitz, AV, Wakefield, JC. (2012): *All We Have to Fear: Psychiatry's Transformation of Natural Anxieties into Mental Disorders*. New York: Oxford University Press.

Hudson, JL Hiripi, E, Pope, HG, Kessler, RC. (2007): The prevalence and correlates of eating disorders in the National Comorbidity Survey Replication. *Biological Psychiatry*, 61: 348–358.

Hyman, S. (2007): Can neuroscience be integrated into the DSM-V? *Nature Reviews Neuroscience*, 8: 725–732.

Hyman, S. (2010): The diagnosis of mental disorders: the problem of reification. *Annual Review of Clinical Psychology*, 6: 155–179.

Hyman, S. (2011): Diagnosis of mental disorders in the light of modern genetics. In Regier, D, Narrow, WE, Kuhl, E, Kupfer, DJ. (Eds.), *The Conceptual Evolution of DSM-5*. Washington, DC: American Psychiatric Publishing, pp. 3–18.

Insel, TR. (2009): A strategic plan for research on mental illness translating scientific opportunity into public health impact. *Archives of General Psychiatry*, 66: 128–133.

Insel, T, Quirion, R. (2005): Psychiatry as a clinical neuroscience discipline. *Journal of the American Medical Association*, 294: 2221–2224.

Ioannidis, JPA. (2005): Why most published research findings are false. *PLoS Med*, 2(8): e124.

Iversen A, Fear NT, Hull L, Greenberg N, Jones M, Browne T, Murphy D, Hotopf M, Rona R, Wessely S. (2007): Pre-enlistment vulnerability factors and their influence on health outcomes amongst UK Military Personnel. *British Journal of Psychiatry*, 191: 506–511.

Jacob, V, Cahttopadhyay, SK, Sipe, TA, Thota, AB, Byard, GJ, Chapman, DP. (2012): Economics of collaborative care for management of depressive disorders: a community guide systematic review. *American Journal of Preventive Medicine*, 42: 539–549.

Jobe, TH, Harrow, M. (2005): Long-term outcome of patients with schizophrenia: a review. *Canadian Journal of Psychiatry*, 50: 892–900.

Kahnemann, D. (2011): *Thinking Fast and Slow*. New York: Macmillan.

Kanner, L. (1943): Autistic disturbances of affective contact. *Nervous Child*, 2: 217–250.

Kendler, KS. (1990): Towards a scientific psychiatric nosology: strengths and limitations. *Archives of General Psychiatry*, 47: 969–973.

Kendler, KS. (2005): "A Gene for…": the nature of gene action in psychiatric disorders. *American Journal of Psychiatry*, 162: 1243–1252.

Kendler, KS, Neale, M, Kessler, R. (1995): The structure of the genetic and environmental risk factors for six major psychiatric disorders in women. *Archives of General Psychiatry*, 52: 474–470.

Kendler, KS, Karkowski, LM, Prescott, CA. (1999): Causal relationship between stressful life events and the onset of major depression. *American Journal of Psychiatry*, 156: 837–841.

Kessler, RC, Adler, L, Barkley, R, Biederman, J, Conners, CK. (2006): The prevalence and correlates of adult ADHD in the United States: results from the National Comorbidity Survey replication. *American Journal of Psychiatry*, 163: 716–723.

Kessler, RC, Anthony, JC, Blazer, DG, Bromet, E, Eaton, WW, Kendler, K, Swartz, M, Wittchen, H-U, Zhao, S. (1997). The US National Comorbidity Survey: overview and future directions. *Epidemiologia e Psichiatria Sociale*, 6: 4–16.

Kessler, RC, Berglund PA, Chu, WT, Deitz, AC, Hudson, JI. (2013): The prevalence and correlates of binge eating disorder in the World Health Organization World Mental Health Surveys. *Biological Psychiatry*, 73: 904–914.

Kessler, RC, Chiu, WT, Demler, O, Merikangas, KR, Walters, EE. (2005a): Prevalence, severity, and comorbidity of 12-month DSM-IV disorders in the National Comorbidity Survey Replication. *Archives of General Psychiatry*, 62: 617–627.

Kessler, RC, Demler, O, Frank, RG, Olfson, M, Pincus, HA, Walters, EE, et al. (2005b): Prevalence and treatment of mental disorders, 1990 to 2003. *New England Journal of Medicine*, 352: 2515–2523.

Kim, YS, Leventhal, BL, Koh, Y-J, Fombonne, E, Laska, EE, Lim, C, et al. (2011): Prevalence of autism spectrum disorders in a total population sample. *American Journal of Psychiatry*, 168: 904–912.

Kirmayer, LJ, Gold, I. (2012): Critical neuroscience and the limits of reductionism. In Choudury, S, Slaby, J (Eds.), *Critical Neuroscience: A Handbook of the Social and Cultural Contexts of Neuroscience*, pp. 307–330. New York: Wiley-Blackwell.

Kirsch, I, Deacon, BJ, Huedo-Medina, TB, Scoboria, A, Moore, TJ. (2008): Initial severity and antidepressant benefits: a meta-analysis of data submitted to the Food and Drug Administration. *PLoS Med*, 5: e45.

Klerman, G. (1986): Historical perspectives on contemporary schools of psychopathology. In Millon, T, Klerman, G (Eds.), *Contemporary Psychopathology: Towards the DSM-IV*. New York: Guilford, pp. 3–28.

Klerman GL. (1990): The psychiatric patient's right to effective treatment: implications of Osheroff v. Chestnut Lodge. *American Journal of Psychiatry*, 147: 409–418.

Koenigsberg, H. (2010). Affective instability: Toward an integration of neuroscience and psychological perspectives. *Journal of Personality Disorders*, 24: 60–82.

Kogan, MD, Blumberg, SJ, Boyle, CA, Perrin, JM. (2009): Prevalence of parent-reported diagnosis of autism spectrum disorder among children in the US, 2007. *Pediatrics*, 124: 2022.

Kraemer, HC, Kupfer, DJ, Clarke, DE, Narrow, WE, Regier, DA. (2012): DSM-5: How reliable Is reliable enough? *American Journal of Psychiatry*, 169: 1.

Kraepelin, E. (1921): *Manic-Depressive Insanity and Paranoia* (Barclay, RM, Trans., Robertson, GM, Ed.). Edinburgh: E and S Livingstone.

Kupfer, DJ, Regier, DA. (2011): Neuroscience, clinical evidence, and the future of psychiatric classification in DSM-5. *American Journal of Psychiatry*, 168: 172–174.

Lai, M-C, Lombardo, MV, Baron-Cohen, S. (2013): Autism. *Lancet* (online)

Lake CR, Hurwitz N. (2006). Schizoaffective disorders are psychotic mood disorders: there are no schizoaffective disorders. *Psychiatry Research*, 143: 255–287.

Lambert M (Ed.). (2013): *Handbook of Psychotherapy and Behavior Change*. New York: Wiley.

Lane, C. (2007): *Shyness*. New Haven, CT: Yale University Press.

Lange, KW, Reichl, S, Lange, KM, Tucha, L, Tucha, O. (2010): The history of attention deficit hyperactivity disorder. *ADHD: Attention Deficit Hyperactivity Disorder*, 2: 241–255.

Leighton, AH. (1959): *My Name Is Legion: The Stirling County Study of Psychiatric Disorder and Sociocultural Environment*. New York: Basic Books.

Lenzenweger, MF, Lane, M, Loranger, AW, Kessler, RC. (2007): DSM-IV Personality Disorders in the National Comorbidity Survey Replication. *Biological Psychiatry*, 62: 553–556.

Leucht, S, Hierl, S, Killsing, W, Dodd, M, Davis, JM. (2012): Putting the efficacy of psychiatric and general medicine medication into perspective: review of meta-analyses. *British Journal of Psychiatry*, 97–106.

Leung, AK, Lemay, JF. (2003): Attention deficit hyperactivity disorder: an update. *Advances in Therapeutics*, 20: 305–318.

Linehan, MM. (1993): *Dialectical Behavior Therapy for Borderline Personality Disorder*. New York: Guilford.

Livesley, WJ, Jang, KL, Vernon, PA. (1998): Phenotypic and genetic structure of traits delineating personality disorder. *Archives of General Psychiatry*, 55: 941–948.

Matson, JL, Williams L. (2013): Differential diagnosis and comorbidity: distinguishing autism from other mental health issues. *Neuropsychiatry*, 3: 233–243.

McFarlane, AC. (1989): The aetiology of post-traumatic morbidity: predisposing, precipitating, and perpetuating factors. *British Journal of Psychiatry*, 154: 221–228.

McGorry PD, Yung AR, Bechdolf A, Amminger P. (2008): Back to the future: predicting and reshaping the course of psychotic disorder. *Archives of General Psychiatry*, 65: 25–27.

McGorry, PD, Nelson, B, Goldstone, S, Yung, A. (2010): Clinical staging: a heuristic and practical strategy for new research and better health and social outcomes for psychotic and related mood disorders. *Canadian Journal of Psychiatry*, 55: 486–497.

McHugh, PR. (2005): *The Mind Has Mountains*. Baltimore, MD: Johns Hopkins Press.

McHugh, PR, Treisman, G. (2007): PTSD: a problematic diagnostic category. *Journal of Anxiety Disorders*, 21: 211–22.

McNally, RJ. (2003). *Remembering Trauma*. Cambridge, MA: Belknap Press/Harvard University Press.

McNally, RJ. (2007): Can we solve the mysteries of the National Vietnam Veterans Readjustment Study? *Journal of Anxiety Disorders*, 21: 192–200.

McNally, RJ. (2009): Can we fix PTSD? *Depression and Anxiety*, 26: 597–600.

McNally, RJ, Breslau, N. (2008): Does virtual trauma cause post-traumatic stress disorder? *American Psychologist*, 63: 282–283.

McPartland, JC, Reichow, B, Volkmar, FR. (2012): Sensitivity and specificity of proposed DSM-5 diagnostic criteria for autism spectrum disorder. *Journal of American Acad Child Adolesc Psychiatry*, 51: 368–383.

McPheeters, M, Warren, Z, Sathe, N J., Bruzek, J, Krishnaswami, S, Jerome, R, Veenstra-VanderWeele, J. (2011): A systematic review of medical treatments for children with autism spectrum disorders. *Pediatrics* online, April 4, 2011.

Menninger, K. (1963). *The Vital Balance: The Life Process in Mental Health and Illness*. New York: Viking Penguin.

Miller, GA. (1956). The magical number seven, plus or minus two. *Psychological Review*, 63: 81–97.

Moffitt, TE, Caspi, A, Marrington, H, Milne, B, Melchior, M, Goldberg, D, et al. (2010): Generalized anxiety disorder and depression: childhood risk factors in a birth cohort followed to 32 years. In Goldberg, D, Kendler, KS, Sirovatka, PJ, Regier, DA (Eds.). *Diagnostic Issues in Depression and Generalized Anxiety Disorder: Refining the Research Agenda for DSM-V*. Washington, DC: American Psychiatric Press, pp. 217–240.

Moffitt, TE, Caspi, A, Taylor, A, Kokaua, J. (2009): How common are common mental disorders? Evidence that lifetime prevalence rates are doubled by prospective versus retrospective ascertainment. *Psychological Medicine*, 40: 899–909.

Mojtabai, R. (2013): Clinician-identified depression in community settings: concordance with structured-interview diagnoses. *Psychotherapy and Psychosomatics*, 82: 161–169.

Mojtabai, R, Olfson, M. (2008): National trends in psychotherapy by office-based psychiatrists. *Archives of General Psychiatry*, 65: 962–970.

Mojtabai, R, Olfson, M. (2010): National trends in psychotropic medication polypharmacy in office-based psychiatry. *Archives of General Psychiatry*, 67: 26–36.

Mojtabai R, Olfson, M. (2011): Proportion of antidepressants prescribed without a psychiatric diagnosis is growing. *Health Affairs*, 30: 1434–1442.

Moncrieff, J, Cohen, D. (2009): How do psychiatric drugs work? *British Medical Journal*, 338: b1963.

Monroe, SM, Simons, AD. (1991): Diathesis-stress theories in the context of life stress research. *Psychological Bulletin*, 110: 406–425.

Morrison, AP, French, P, Stewart, SL, Birchwood, M. (2012): Early detection and intervention evaluation for people at risk of psychosis: multisite randomised controlled trial. *British Medical Journal*, 344: e2233.

Moynihan, R, Heath, I, Henry, D. (2002): Selling sickness: the pharmaceutical industry and disease mongering. *British Medical Journal*, 324: 886–891.

National Institute for Health and Clinical Excellence (2009): *Depression: management of depression in primary and secondary care*. Accessed online, June 2012.

Newton-Howes, G, Tyrer, P, Johnson, T. (2006). Personality disorder and the outcome of depression: meta-analysis of published studies. *British Journal of Psychiatry*, 188: 13–20.

North, CS, Suris, AM, Davis, D., Smith, RP. (2009): Toward validation of the diagnosis of Posttraumatic Stress Disorder. *American Journal of Psychiatry*, 166: 34–41.

166 | REFERENCES

Offer, D., Sabshin, M. (1966): *Normality; theoretical and clinical concepts of mental health*. New York: Basic Books.

Olfson, M, Blanco, C, Wang, S, Greenhill, LL. (2013): Trends in office-based treatment of adults with stimulants in the United States. *Journal of Clinical Psychiatry*, 74: 43–50.

Pacheco-Unguetti, AP, Acosta, A, Callejas, A, Lupianez J. (2010): Attention and anxiety: different attentional functioning under state and trait anxiety. *Psychological Science*, 21: 298–304.

Palmer, BA, Pankrantz, VS, Bostwick, JM. (2005): The lifetime risk of suicide in schizophrenia: a reexamination. *Archives of General Psychiatry*, 62: 247–253.

Parens, E, Johnstone, J. (2009): Facts, values, and Attention-Deficit Hyperactivity Disorder (ADHD): an update on the controversies. *Child and Adolescent Psychiatry and Mental Health*, 3: 1–10.

Paris, J. (2008a): *Prescriptions for the Mind*. New York: Oxford University Press.

Paris, J. (2008b): *Treatment of Borderline Personality Disorder: A Guide to Evidence-Based Practice*. New York: Guilford Press.

Paris, J. (2010a): The Use and Misuse of Psychiatric Drugs: An Evidence-Based Critique. London: John Wiley.

Paris, J. (2010c): Estimating the prevalence of personality disorders. *Journal of Personality Disorders*, 24: 405–411.

Paris, J. (2010d): Effectiveness of differing psychotherapy approaches in the treatment of borderline personality disorder. *Current Psychiatry Reports*, 12: 56–60.

Paris, J. (2012): *The Bipolar Spectrum: Diagnosis or Fad?* New York: Routledge.

Paris, J. (2012b): The rise and fall of dissociative disorders. *Journal of Nervous and Mental Diseases*, 200: 1076–1079.

Paris, J. (2013): *The Intelligent Clinician's Guide to DSM-5*. New York: Oxford University Press.

Paris, J. (2013a): *The Intelligent Clinician's Guide to DSM-5*. New York: Oxford University Press.

Paris, J. (2013b): *Fads and Fallacies in Psychiatry*. London: Royal College of Psychiatrists.

Paris, J. (2013c): The limits of phenomenology. *Acta Psychiatric Scandinavica*, 128: 384.

Paris, J, Phillips, J, eds. (2013): *Making DSM-5: Historical, Ideological, and Conceptual Issues in the DSM Process*. New York: Springer.

Parker, G. (2005): Beyond major depression. *Psychological Medicine*, 35: 467–474.

Parker, G. (2011): Classifying clinical depression: an operational proposal. *Acta Psychiatrica Scandinavica*, 123: 314–316.

Parker, G. (2012): *Bipolar-II Disorder. Modelling, Measuring and Managing* (2nd ed.). Cambridge, UK: Cambridge University Press.

Parker, G, Fletcher, K, Hadzi-Pavlovic, D. (2011): Is context everything to the definition of clinical depression? A test of the Horwitz and Wakefield postulate, *Journal of Affective Disorders*, 136: 1034–1038.

Patten, SB. (2008): Major depression prevalence is high, but the syndrome is a poor proxy for community populations' clinical needs. *Canadian Journal of Psychiatry*, 53: 411–419.

Perugi, G, Angst, J, Azorin J-M, Bowden, C, Vieta, E, Young, AH. (2013): The bipolar-borderline personality disorders connection in major depressive patients. *Acta Psychiatric Scandinavica*, 128: 376–383.

Pope, HG, Lipinski, JR. (1978): Diagnosis in schizophrenia and manic-depressive illness: a reassessment of the specificity of 'schizophrenic' symptoms in the light of current research. *Archives of General Psychiatry*, 35: 811–828.

Posner, MI. (2012). *Attention in a Social World*. New York: Oxford University Press.

Posternak, MA, Zimmerman, M. (2005): Is there a delay in the antidepressant effect? A meta-analysis. *Journal of Clinical Psychiatry*, 66: 148–158.

Pratt, LA, Brody, DJ, Gu, Q. (2011): *Antidepressant use in persons aged 12 and over: United States, 2005–2008*. NCHS data brief, no 76. Hyattsville, MD: National Center for Health Statistics.

Razali, SM. (2000): Masked depression: an ambiguous diagnosis. *Australian and New Zealand Journal of Psychiatry*, 34(1): 167–170.

Rapoport, JI, Buchsbaum, MS, Zahn, TP, Weingartner, H, Ludlow, C, Mikkelsen EJ. (1978): Dextroamphetamine: cognitive and behavioral effects in normal prepubertal boys. *Science*, 199: 560–563.

Rauch, SAM, Eftekhari, A, Ruzek, JI. (2012): Review of exposure therapy: a gold standard for PTSD treatment. *Journal of Rehabilitation Research and Development*, 49: 679–688.

Regier, DA, Narrow, WE, Clarke, DE, Kraekere, HC, Kuramoto, J, Kuhl EA, Kupfer, DJ. (2013): DSM-5 Field Trials in the United States and Canada, Part II: test-retest reliability of selected categorical diagnoses. *American Journal of Psychiatry*, 170: 59–70.

Robins, E, Guze, SB. (1970): Establishment of diagnostic validity in psychiatric illness: its application to schizophrenia. *American Journal of Psychiatry*, 126: 107–111.

Robins, L. (1966): *Deviant Children Grown Up*. Baltimore, MD: Williams and Wilkins.

Robins LN, Regier DA. (1991): *Psychiatric Disorders in America*. New York: Free Press.

Rosen, GM, Lilienfeld, SO. (2008): Post-traumatic stress disorder: an empirical evaluation of core assumptions. *Clinical Psychology Review*, 28: 837–868.

Ruggero, C, Zimmerman, M, Chelminski, I, Young, D. (2010): Borderline personality disorder and the misdiagnosis of bipolar disorder. *Journal of Psychiatric Research*, 44: 405–408.

Russell, G. (1979): Bulimia nervosa: an ominous variant of anorexia nervosa *Psychological Medicine*, 9: 429–448.

Rutter, M, Uher, R. (2012): Classification issues and challenge in child and adolescent psychiatry. *International Review of Psychiatry*, 24: 514–529.

Satel S, Lillienfeld, S. (2013): *Brainwashed: The Seductive Appeal of Mindless Neuroscience*. New York: Basic Books.

Schneider, K. (1959): *Clinical Psychopathology*. New York: Grune and Stratton.

Schou, M. (2001). Lithium treatment at 52. *Journal of Affective Disorders*, 67: 21–32.

Seidler, GH, Wagner, FE. (2006): Comparing the efficacy of EMDR and trauma-focused cognitive-behavioral therapy in the treatment of PTSD: a meta-analytic study. *Psychological Medicine*, 36: 1515–1522.

Shah, PJ, Morton, MJS. (2013): Attention deficit hyperactivity disorder: diagnosis or normality? *British Journal of Psychiatry*, 203: 317–319.

Sharma, V, Khan, M, Smith, A. (2005): A closer look at treatment resistant depression: is it due to a bipolar diathesis? *Journal of Affective Disorders*, 84: 251–257.

Shorter, E. (1997): *A History of Psychiatry: From the Era of the Asylum to the Age of Prozac.* New York: John Wiley & Sons.

Shorter, E. (2008): *Before Prozac: The Troubled History of Mood Disorders in Psychiatry.* New York: Oxford University Press.

Siever, LJ. (2007): Biologic factors in schizotypal personality disorders. *Acta Psychiatrica Scandinavica,* 90: 45–50.

Siever, LJ, Davis, KL. (1991): A psychobiological perspective on the personality disorders. *American Journal of Psychiatry,* 148: 1647–1658.

Singh, I. (2008): Beyond polemics: science and ethics of ADHD. *Nature Reviews Neuroscience,* 9: 957–964.

Skodol, AE. (2010): Dimensionalizing existing personality disorder categories. In Millon, T, Krueger, R, Simonsen, E (Eds.), *Contemporary Directions in Psychopathology: Scientific foundations of the DSM-V and ICD-11.* New York: Guilford Press, pp. 372–373.

Skodol, AE, Bender, DS, Morey, LM, Clark, LA, Oldham, J, Alarcon, RD, et al. (2011a). Personality disorder types proposed for DSM-5. *Journal of Personality Disorders,* 25: 137–142.

Skodol, AE, Grilo, CM, Keyes, KM, Geier, T, Grant, BF, Hasin, DS. (2011b): Relationship of personality disorders to the course of major depressive disorder in a nationally representative sample. *American Journal of Psychiatry,* 168: 257–264.

Spitzer, RL. (1976): More on pseudoscience in science and the case for psychiatric diagnosis. *Archives of General Psychiatry,* 33: 459–470.

Srole, L, Fischer, AK. (1980): The Midtown Manhattan Longitudinal Study vs. "The Mental Paradise Lost Doctrine." *Archives of General Psychiatry,* 37: 209–218.

Starkevic, M, Portman, M. (2013): The status quo as a good outcome: how the DSM-5 diagnostic criteria for generalized anxiety disorder remained unchanged from the DSM-IV criteria. *Australia and New Zealand Journal of Psychiatry* online. doi:0004867413503719.

Stoffers, J, Völlm, BA, Rücker, G, Timmer, A, Huband, N, Lieb, K. (2012). Pharmacological interventions for borderline personality disorder. *Cochrane Database of Systematic Reviews,* issue 6: CD005653. doi:10.1002/14651858.CD005653.pub2.

Stoffers, JM, Völlm, BA, Rücker, G, Timmer, A, Huband, N, Lieb, K. (2012b): Psychological therapies for people with borderline personality. *Cochrane Database of Systematic Reviews*, issue 8, CD005652.

Taylor, MA. (2013): *Hippocrates Cried: The Decline of American Psychiatry*. New York: Oxford University Press.

Thombs, BD, de Jonge, P, Coyne, JC, Whooley, MA. (2008): Depression screening and patient outcomes in cardiovascular care: a systematic review. *Journal of the American Medical Association*, 300: 2161–2171.

Thompson, T. (2013): Autism research and services for young children: history, progress and challenges. *Journal of Applied Research in Intellectual Disabilities*, 26: 81–107.

Trull, TJ, Jahng, S, Tomko, RL, Wood, PK, Sher, KJ. (2010): Revised NESARC personality disorder diagnoses: gender, prevalence, and comorbidity with substance dependence disorders. *Journal of Personality Disorders*, 24: 412–426.

Uher, R, Rutter, M. (2012): Basing psychiatric classification on scientific foundation: problems and prospects. *International Review of Psychiatry*, 24: 591–605.

Valenstein, M. (2006): Keeping our eyes on STAR*D. *American Journal of Psychiatry*, 193: 1484–1486.

Van Os, J. (2009): 'Salience syndrome' replaces 'schizophrenia' in DSM-V and ICD-11: Psychiatry's evidence-based entry into the 21st century? *Acta Psychiatrica Scandinavica*, 120: 363–372.

Wakefield, JC. (2007): What makes a mental disorder mental? *Philosophy, Psychiatry, and Psychology*, 13: 123–131.

Wakefield, JC, Schmitz, MF, First, MB, Horwitz, A. (2007): Extending the bereavement exclusion for major depression to other losses. *Archives of General Psychiatry*, 64: 433–440.

Wakefield, JC. (2012): DSM-5: proposed changes to depressive disorders. *Current Medical Research & Opinion*, 28: 335–343.

Weiss, G, Hechtman, L. (2002): *Hyperactive Children Grown Up: ADHD in Children, Adolescents, and Adults* (2nd ed.). New York: Guilford.

Welch, HG, Schwartz, L, Woloshin, S. (2011): *Overdiagnosed: Making People Sick in the Pursuit of Health*. Boston: Beacon Press.

Wittchen, H-U, Fehm, L. (2001): Epidemiology, patterns of comorbidity, and associated disabilities of social phobia. *Psychiatric Clinics of North America*, 24: 617–641.

Young, A. (1997): *The Harmony of Illusions: Inventing Post-Traumatic Stress Disorder.* Princeton, NJ: Princeton University Press.

Young, AH, Hammond, JM. (2007): Lithium in mood disorders: increasing evidence base, declining use? *British Journal of Psychiatry*, 191: 474–476.

Zanarini, MC, Gunderson, JG, Frankenburg, FR, Chauncey, DL. (1989): The Revised Diagnostic Interview for Borderlines: discriminating BPD from other Axis II disorders. *Journal of Personality Disorders*, 3: 10–18.

Zanarini, MC, Frankenburg, F, Reich, B, Fitzmaurice, G. (2012): Attainment and stability of sustained symptomatic remission and recovery among borderline patients and Axis II comparison subjects: a 16-year prospective followup study. *American Journal of Psychiatry*, 169: 476–483.

Zimmerman, M, Chelminski, I. (2003): Generalized anxiety disorder in patients with major depression: is DSM-IV's hierarchy correct? *American Journal of Psychiatry*, 160: 504–512.

Zimmerman, M, Chelminski, I, Young, D, Dalyrymple, K, Martinez, J. (2011): Does DSM-IV already capture the dimensional nature of personality disorders? *Journal of Clinical Psychiatry.* doi:10.4088/JCP.11m06974.

Zimmerman, M, Chelminski, I, Young D, Dalyrymple, K, Martinez, J. (2012): Impact of deleting 5 DSM-IV personality disorders on prevalence, comorbidity, and the association between personality disorder pathology and psychosocial morbidity. *Journal of Clinical Psychiatry*, 73: 202–207.

Zimmerman, M, Dalrymple, K, Chelminski, I, Young, D, Galione, JN. (2010): Recognition of irrationality of fear and the diagnosis of social anxiety disorders and specific phobia in adults" implications for criteria revision in DSM-5. *Depression & Anxiety*, 27: 1044–1049.

Zimmerman, M, Galione, J. (2010): Psychiatrists' and nonpsychiatrist physicians' reported use of the DSM-IV criteria for major depressive disorder. *Journal of Clinical Psychiatry*, 71: 235–238.

Zimmerman, M, Galione, JN, Ruggero, CJ, Chelminski, I, Young, D, Dalrymple, K, McGlinchey, JB. (2010): Screening for bipolar disorder and finding borderline personality disorder. *Journal of Clinical Psychiatry*, 71: 1212–1217.

Zimmerman, M, Mattia, J. (1999): Differences between clinical and research practices in diagnosing borderline personality disorder. *American Journal of Psychiatry*, 156: 1570–1574.

Zimmerman, M, Rothschild, L, Chelminski, I. (2005). The prevalence of DSM-IV personality disorders in psychiatric outpatients. *American Journal of Psychiatry*, 162: 1911–1918.

Zimmerman, M, Thongy, T. (2007): How often do SSRIs and other new-generation antidepressants lose their effect during continuation treatment? Evidence suggesting the rate of true tachyphylaxis during continuation treatment is low. *Journal of Clinical Psychiatry*, 68: 1271–1276.

Zohar, J, Fostick, L, Cohen, A, Bleich, A, Dolfin, D, Weissman, Z, Doron, M, Kaplan, Z, Klein, E, Shalev, A. (2009): Risk factors for the development of posttraumatic stress disorder following combat trauma: a semiprospective study. *Journal of Clinical Psychiatry*, 70: 1629–1635.

Zorumski, R. (2009): Looking forward. In North, CS, Yutzy, SH. (Eds.), *Goodwin and Guze's Psychiatric Diagnosis*. New York: Oxford University Press, pp. xxv–xxxii.

Zorumski C, Rubin E. (2011): *Psychiatry and Clinical Neuroscience: A Primer*. New York: Oxford University Press.

INDEX

Made in the USA
Coppell, TX
21 October 2020